OPERATION *cleanse*

Indhira Santana, CNHP, MBA, HHC
& Violet Santana, ND, CNHP

First published in 2017 by Indhira Santana and Violet Santana

ISBN 978-0-9855724-4-0

Disclaimer:
The contents of this book are intended to help you make informed health decisions, not replace, any treatment prescribed by your medical doctor. If you are aware, or suspect, that you have a health problem, you should consult your medical doctor. In the event you use any of the information in this book, the authors disclaim any responsibility incurred as a consequence of the use of this information.

Printed in the USA

Book Design by Danielle Mehta

Photography by Indhira Santana and Violet Santana

dedication

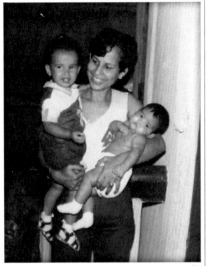

Dominican Republic, 1985

To our mom, Hilda,

This book is for you. We are forever thankful for your immeasurable strength, wisdom, and desire to help others. It's because of you that we strive to make this world a healthier and happier place. Thank you for being such a great role model and for always pushing us to be better than we were yesterday.

Por ti, estamos agradecidas.

Indhira & Violet

Contents

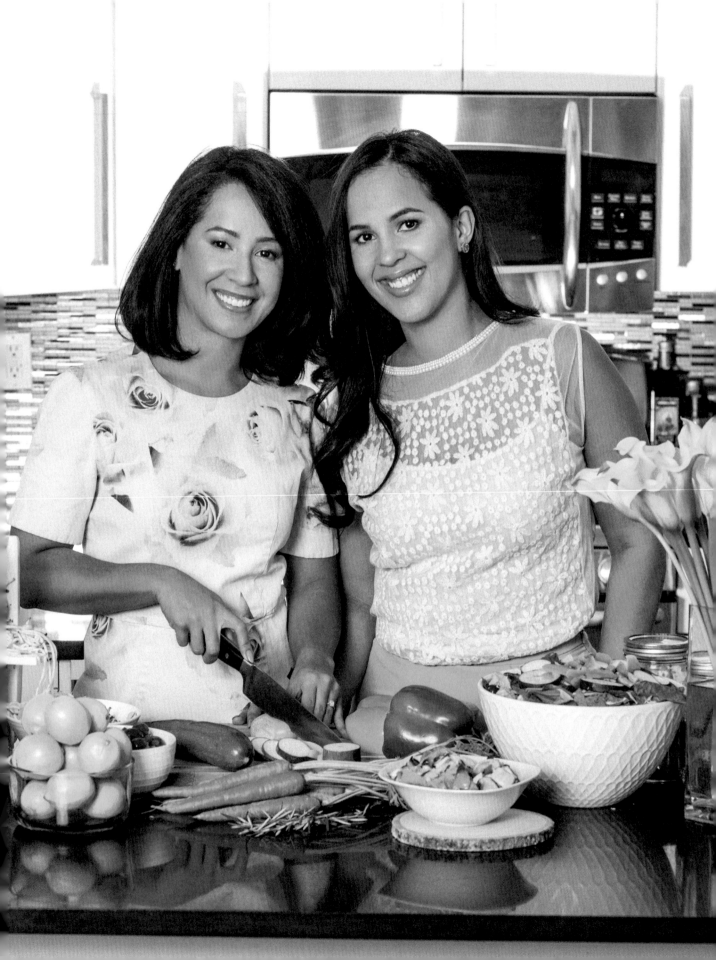

A MESSAGE FROM

Indhira & Violet Santana

We hope that you are as excited about starting Operation Cleanse as we are to help you on your detox journey. If you commit yourself, stay open to trying new things, and most importantly be willing to leave those bad food habits in the past, we promise that this will be the most amazing 14 days of your life.

Operation Cleanse is exactly what we wished we had at our disposal as we dealt with our own health issues. Indhira was overweight, unhappy and always trying a new diet. The result of said diets was that the weight always came back. Although Violet never dealt with weight issues, her sugar and carb addiction led her to suffer from what we call "skinny sick". Her list of issues included psoriasis all over the body, year-long allergies, almost monthly yeast (candida) infections and at one point, a weakened immune system leading to five colds in one year.

It took us years to understand that our symptoms were not the problem; they were simply signs from our bodies letting us know it was time for a fresh start. Like you, we overloaded our bodies with toxic eating, toxic drinking and even toxic thoughts. All these toxins were the root of our problems. We created Operation Cleanse as the solution to detox our bodies.

Operation Cleanse is based on the idea that by cleansing, you give your body the reset it needs to naturally heal itself, rid itself of excess weight and inflammation and give you the energy you need to live your best life. You can achieve this by replacing processed foods with nutritious, whole foods and quality herbs and supplements.

To date, hundreds of our clients have successfully completed Operation Cleanse and pledged to continue living a healthy lifestyle. We hope that you use this as a launch pad to live your best and healthiest life.

In Good Health,
Indhira & Violet

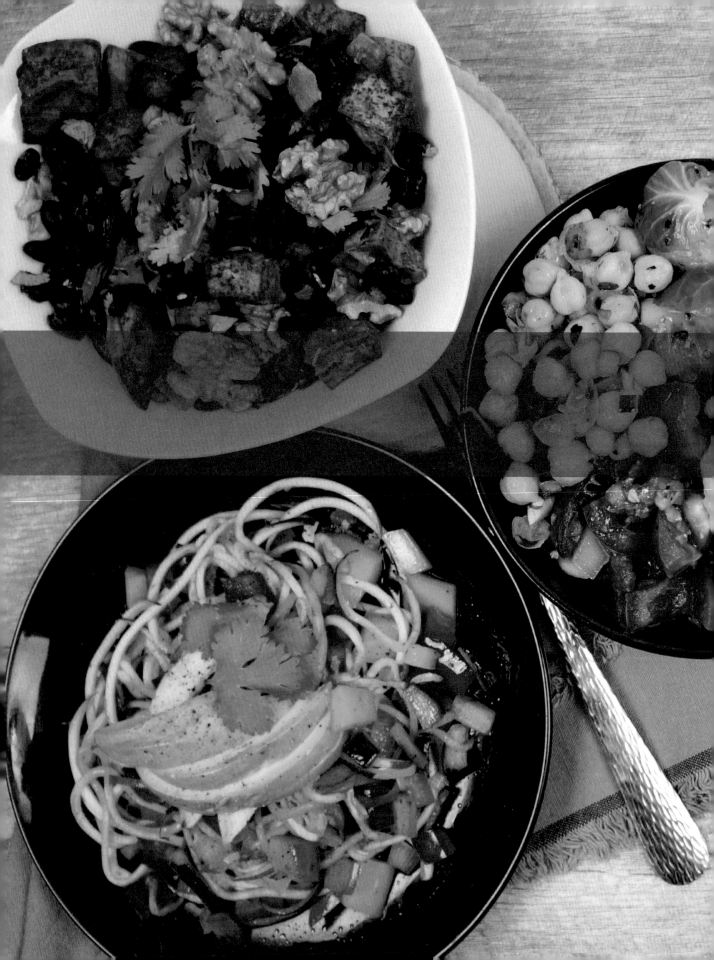

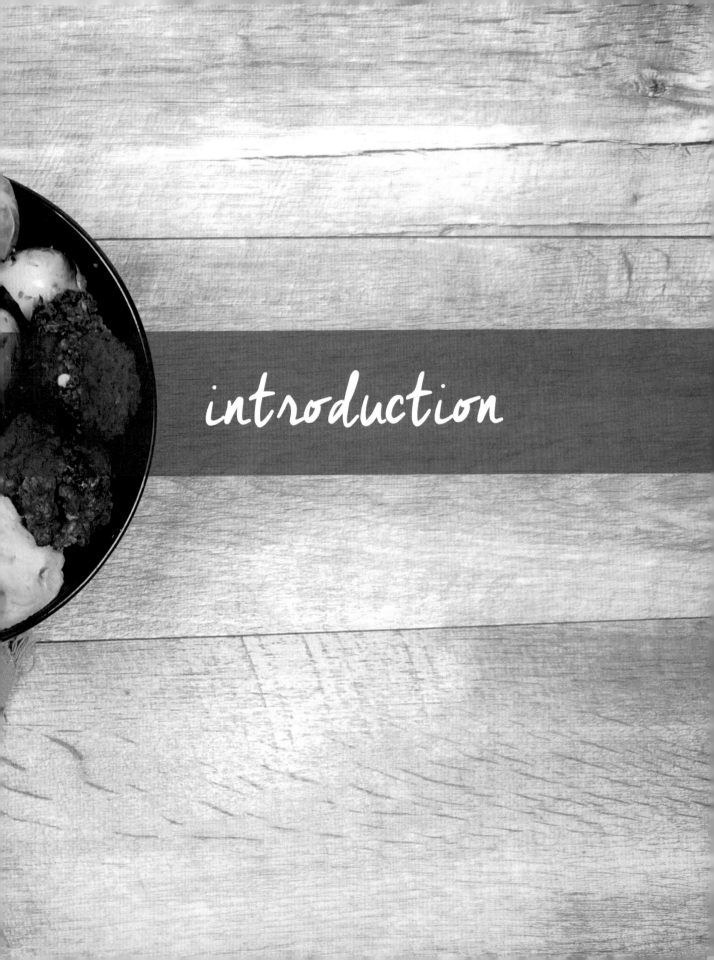

introduction

Reasons to Detox

If you're reading this book, chances are you are ready to feel your best. Throughout this book, you'll find we use the words detox and cleansing interchangeably. There are countless reasons why you should wipe the slate clean internally. Here are the most popular reasons we, and our clients, have:

F.L.C. SYNDROME (FEEL LIKE CRAP)

When our body is overloaded with chemicals and toxins from a crappy diet, we start to feel like crap. Processed, packaged foods are loaded with preservatives, colorants and other chemicals to extend shelf life and maintain texture and taste for extended periods of time. Our bodies are not designed to process these chemicals 365 days a year. Our body does what it can to keep us functioning at full capacity. But, what happens when one organ becomes tired or congested? Other parts of our body pick up the slack and the domino effect begins leading to F.L.C. syndrome.

SUGAR CRAVINGS

A sugar craving is one food addiction we, and many of our clients, struggle with. When you crave sweets and even bread, rice or pasta every day, consider yourself a sugar addict. Here's the bottom line: if you want to take complete control of your health, you need to control your sugar intake. There is no magic advice here. All it takes is dedication, a burning desire to change and some serious self-control.

We know, we know, you "can't" function without those sweet snacks. It's a real addiction. A study performed on lab rats found that Oreo cookies were just as enticing as cocaine due to the similar "feel good" hormones it produces in your brain (we can't make this stuff up if we tried. Go on, Google it!). Now we ask you, if you know it's a real addiction, why are you not doing everything you can to kick that habit?

The good news: sugar cravings are completely natural. They are how your body tells you to give it some energy. It's up to you to feed those cravings with natural sugars as much as possible. That's where Operation Cleanse comes in. You will learn to focus on a diet that is rich in naturally sweet foods to avoid cravings, find sustained energy, and avoid the highs and lows you feel when you swing from processed, refined food to processed, refined food.

WEIGHT LOSS

Think about this...fat cells do many things inside our bodies, including cushioning our organs and keeping us warm. They also trap and store toxicity, lots of it. The greater the amount of fat cells you're carrying around, the more toxicity you're holding on to. Detoxing the body means giving your body the best chance for weight loss. When your body doesn't have to waste energy figuring out what to do with the chemicals from processed food, it can tackle weight loss more effortlessly.

DIGESTIVE PROBLEMS

From constipation, to bloating and acid reflux. Living with just one of these symptoms, day after day, not only leaves you feeling uncomfortable, but slowly stresses your internal organs. Constipation for example, increases the toxic load of the colon. Once it becomes too much for the colon to deal with, the liver, kidneys and even lungs (yes, that foul breath is from constipation) get involved to help dilute the toxic load of the body.

Fact!

Constipation is not only straining, it's also defined as skipping one or more days, having hard stools or feeling like you had an incomplete movement.

CHRONIC SKIN ISSUES

Most of us obsess over what we see in the mirror. What we tend to forget is that the moment we see something off with our skin, weeks and months of inner turmoil have already passed. The skin is considered the largest organ of the body and a key detoxifying organ at that. Cleansing the body internally means less acne, eczema, psoriasis and other skin issues externally.

The Benefits of Cleansing

We can write an entire book on just the benefits of cleansing your body, but we'd rather share the key benefits our clients have experienced during their time at My Wellness Solutions and as participants of Operation Cleanse.

INCREASED ENERGY

Few things in life can beat the feeling of waking up refreshed and naturally energized. No, we don't mean a caffeinated rush. We mean the increased energy boost you get when your machine (aka your body) is fueled by the pure power of whole foods. You will finally sleep through the night and wake up with a bounce in your step. Goodbye 2PM coffee-break!

CLEARER, BRIGHTER SKIN

When your friends and family start commenting on how great you look, you can thank your glowing skin for that. It's the first thing most people notice when they see you after you complete this cleanse. Operation Cleanse fuels your skin with essential nutrients that help detoxify the skin from the inside out while helping to replenish and generate healthier skin cells.

GOODBYE ALLERGIES

It doesn't matter what your trigger is – dogs, cats, pollen, dust or even food allergies and food sensitivities – the recipes in this book will give your body the much needed boost to your immune system that you've been looking for. The moment your immune system takes a break from battling the toxicity produced from eating fast, processed foods, it can turn its attention to building a stronger, healthier immune system with soldiers ready for whatever life brings your way.

MENTAL CLARITY

Many of us go from a stressful job to a stressful household and nowhere in the middle do we stop to take a mental break. Add a crappy diet on top and it's no wonder we live in a mental fog! You forget where you put your glasses when they were sitting on top of your head the whole time. A top benefit of cleansing and giving the body a break from processed foods is that you gain back the mental focus you thought you left back in your "younger days".

REDUCED INFLAMMATION

Swollen ankles, chronically sore joints and puffy eyes are just a few of the symptoms you can say "SO LONG" to after Operation Cleanse. Whether it's your morning smoothie or your lunchtime dish, all of our recipes will load your body with alkaline rich foods and reduce the toxic load from acid producing foods. Acid foods include processed meats, sweets, refined carbohydrates, alcohol, dairy and sweetened beverages. Alkaline foods include all veggies, fruits, whole grains like quinoa, and water. An alkaline body means a body free of chronic inflammation.

BETTER BOWEL MOVEMENTS

Reality Check: If you do not have at least 1 bowel movement a day or pass painful, small hard stools at any point, you suffer from constipation. Your bowel movements should be abundant and easy to pass. During and after Operation Cleanse, you will experience what a diet high in fiber and water will do to keep your bowel movements happening at least once per day.

According to the U.S. Dept. of Health and Human Services (2016) 63 million Americans suffer from chronic constipation. The culprit? The Standard American Diet (SAD) which provides less than 10 grams of fiber per day when men and women up to 50 years old require 38 grams and 25 grams, respectively.

If this was you prior to Operation Cleanse, the consistency of your bowel movements will change.

Having regular bowel movements is one of the most important goals you should want to achieve and maintain. Having irregular bowel movements makes us sluggish, gives us dull skin, fogs our brain, causes cravings and keeps us overweight. We can keep going with this list but you get the point. Regular cleansing of your colon (even if you do not suffer from constipation) is important to keep all your other organs working optimally as they all work together.

IMPROVED HYDRATION

Forget 8-10 cups of water per day. A person that weighs 220 lbs. requires a different amount of water than the person who weighs 140 lbs. The general rule is that the amount of water your body needs is half your body weight in ounces (ie. if you weigh 220 lbs., divide by half and you get 110. Your body needs 110 oz. of water per day – 10-15% more if you are sweating or working out). From the Operation Cleanse smoothies and the fruits and vegetables high in water content found in the approved recipes, your body is well on it's way to improved hydration.

So...what are people saying?

I lost about 8 lbs. and I'm extremely happy with the results. Yes, the results were unexpected. Thanks so much!! The Facebook chat and emails helped me stay on track knowing that other people were doing the same thing I was and they were keeping up with it.

- Jennifer Roman, NY -

I lost 9 lbs. Yes! I'm so excited. I learned so much on eating healthy with yummy foods :) It was unexpected in the sense that I was still eating and drinking shakes and still managed to lose the weight.

- Annette Barraza, NY -

I lost 7 lbs. I didn't go into it expecting to lose much weight just because of past experience and my health issues which make it difficult. This was a pleasant surprise. I feel better than I've felt in a VERY long time and that makes me want to keep focused on making healthy living a lifelong thing. Thanks for the push and willingness to help people like me embark on something so necessary.

- Sasha Palin, NJ -

BREAKING UP WITH ALCOHOL, GLUTEN, DAIRY & SUGAR

Let's be honest for a moment, a glass of wine paired with cheese and crackers can be a hard one to break up with – even for 14 days. But to get the results you want, you should get ready to see what life is like without these substances overloading your body – alcohol, gluten, sugar and dairy. Yes, it will be a messy breakup, but your "post cleanse self" will thank you for it. Here's why.

ALCOHOL

Even small amounts of alcohol can alter the liver detoxification process that we activate during the cleanse with our food and supplements. Alcohol stresses the liver and slows down its detox process. So, say no to booze!

GLUTEN

For the purpose of this cleanse we're eliminating gluten. Gluten is the protein that helps wheat products stick together – and it can create a sticky mess inside our gut too. Gluten usually comes in foods that we'll be avoiding anyway – breads, biscuits, pasta, etc. It's often poorly tolerated by our digestive system, and can be inflammatory to pre-existing conditions like allergies and bloating.

DAIRY

Aside from being highly acidic and full of hormones, dairy and lactose in particular can be difficult to digest. It also contributes to excess mucus formation in the body. If you have allergies, dairy can exacerbate these problems. Replace dairy with almond milk, rice milk, or coconut milk.

SUGAR

What else can we say besides, goodbye sugar? During the Sugar Detox phase, you will eliminate processed sugar (and even starchy vegetables and many fruits). This will be the most challenging aspect of the cleanse for many of you so make sure you check back with your intentions often and pay close attention to how you address your cravings.

There are two important things to remember about "clean eating"

FIRST

You need to make it work for your body. Not everyone's digestion can (or should) handle a raw vegan diet, nor will everyone flourish on a diet rich in whole grains and legumes. It's about finding what works for you!

SECOND

You need to make it sustainable for your lifestyle. There's no point in creating a huge meal plan with elaborate recipes if you don't have time to make them. Perhaps you don't love cooking and need simple meals that can be prepped ahead of time (most of our recipes are simple). Or you have limited space and appliances, or maybe you don't have access to fresh organic produce on a weekly basis. Whatever your situation, there's a way that you can make healthy eating work for you and your family. Regardless of the situation, you should ALWAYS make time for your health.

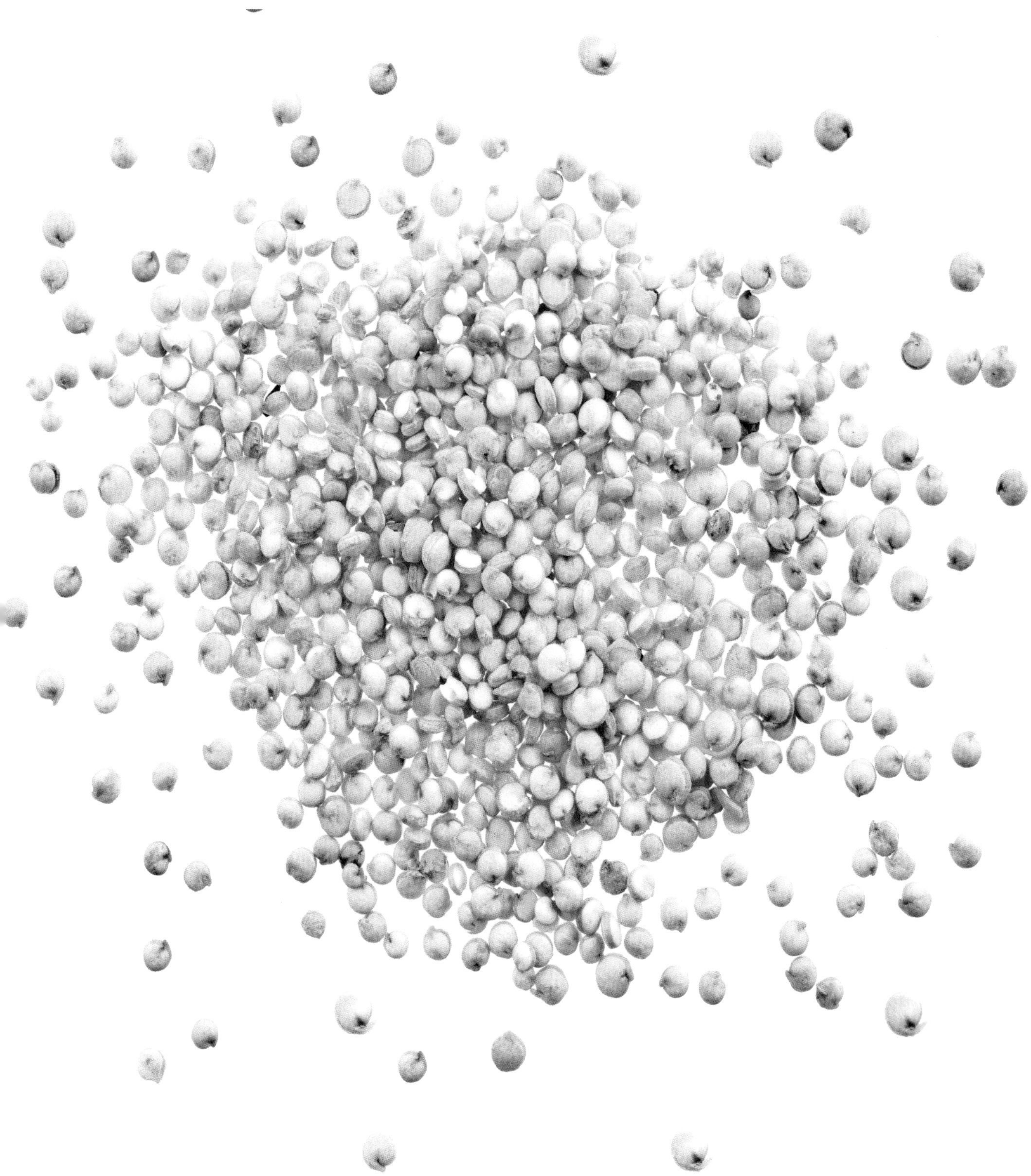

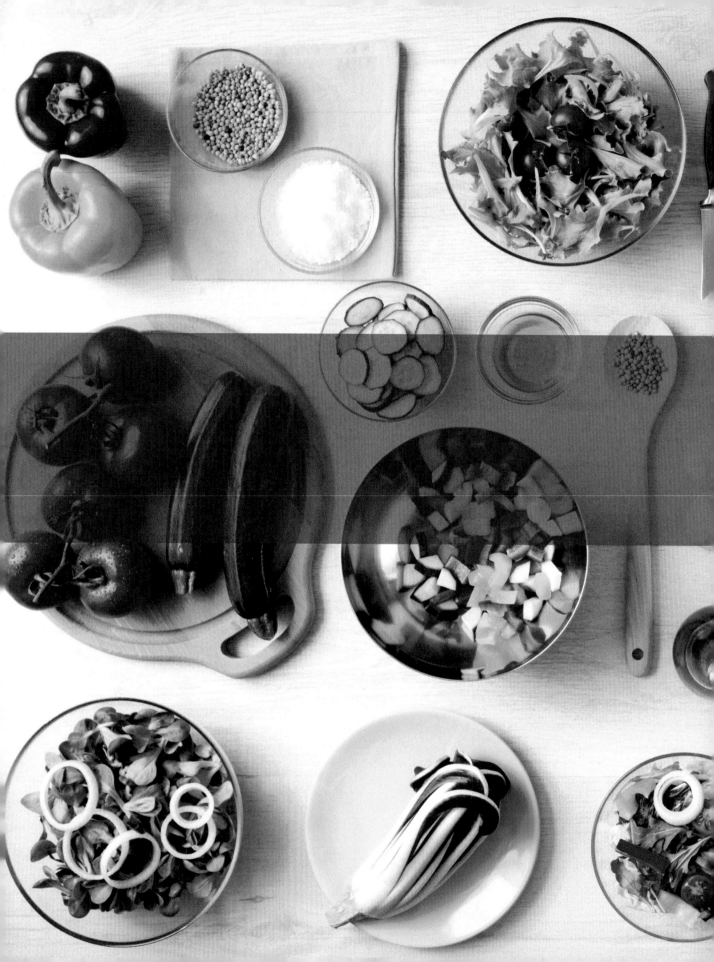

PART 1 | *the details*

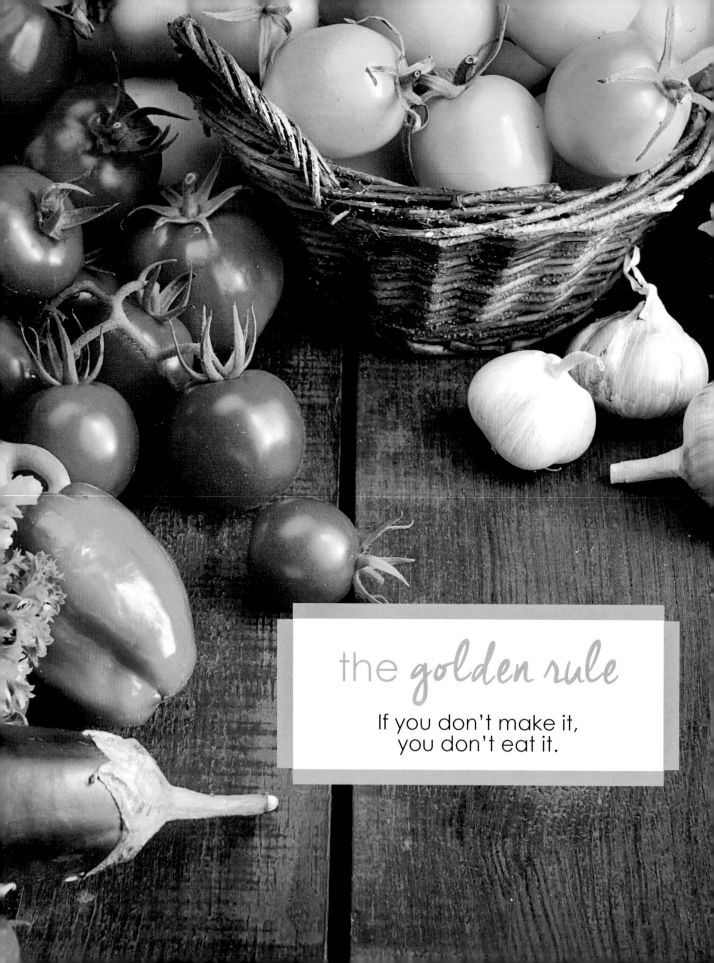

the *golden rule*

If you don't make it,
you don't eat it.

How to Operation Cleanse

Operation Cleanse is based on the principle that by eating the right food combinations, you support your body as it cleanses itself of the toxins wearing you out. During this cleanse you will eat foods that are whole, nutrient- rich, and cooked by you. The most important thing to keep in mind is that this program isn't about deprivation or eating boring foods – we've filled this book with the most popular recipes from our previous programs in which thousands of our clients rated as tasty, flavorful, and most important, easy to make!

Operation Cleanse is designed as a 3-step process to help you optimize whatever health results you desire. Read this entire section before skipping to the recipes and sample menus.

STEP 1 - THE PRE-CLEANSE

To start preparing your body for what's to come, it's CRUCIAL that you pre-cleanse. This phase lasts 4-5 days and is when you start to taper down on addictive substances like caffeine, dairy (yes, cheese too), sugar and alcohol.

STEP 2 - THE CLEANSE

During the cleanse, you follow a 14-day routine broken down into two parts: 7 days of Vegan Detox and 7 days of Sugar Detox. During this time, you follow a simple meal plan that consists of smoothies, whole foods, delicious snacks and quality supplements.

Vegan Detox
The 7-day Vegan Detox helps you determine which foods may be the cause of symptoms like chronic bloating and constipation. You will incorporate a vegan diet and explore alternative sources to animal proteins.

Sugar Detox
During the 7-day Sugar Detox we tackle those sugar addictions by eliminating foods that your body quickly turns into sugar (aka glucose). That includes high glycemic fruits and even beans and root vegetables.

STEP 3 - THE RE-INTRODUCTION

After your 14-day cleanse, the re-introduction phase is where you begin to understand what foods serve you and which don't. By reintroducing foods back into your diet as we've suggested post Operation Cleanse, you will learn your food intolerances and sensitivities so you can live a life free of bloating, constipation, and any other symptoms that troubled you.

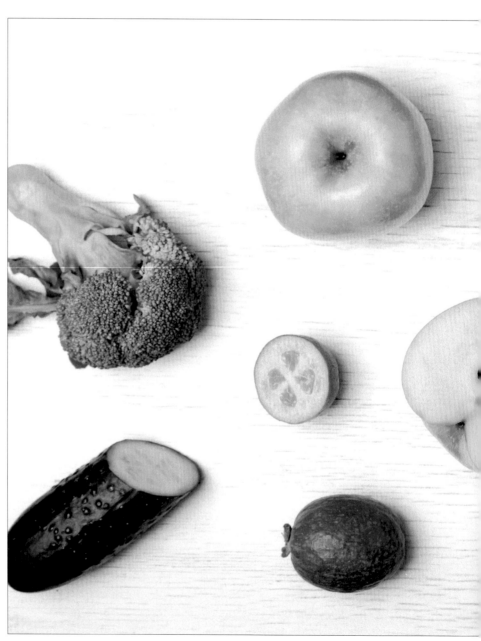

The "No" List

During the entire 14-day cleanse, eliminate the following completely.

All processed, refined, factory-made foods. If you don't make it, don't eat it. No exceptions!

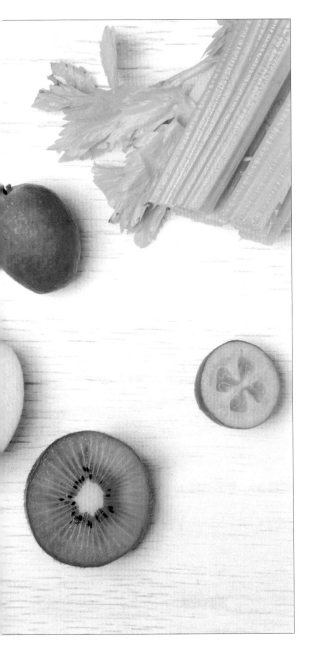

- Caffeine – including caffeinated teas
- Alcohol
- Dairy – including all cow milk, yogurt and all cheeses
- Gluten
- All processed drinks including fruit juices, sodas and "natural" juices that come from a supermarket
- All refined and processed vegetable oils (goodbye corn and canola oil!)
- Other stimulants – if you are a smoker, take a break during this time also

check it out!

What's allowed
and what's not...

The "Yes" List

	ALLOWED	NOT ALLOWED
Fruits	All fresh fruits except those in the not allowed list	Grapes, bananas, dried fruits, canned fruits, frozen fruits
Green Vegetables	All green vegetables	
Starchy Vegetables	Vegan Detox: Butternut squash, sweet potatoes, acorn squash	Sugar Detox: ALL starchy vegetables including corn, potatoes, plantains, casava, yucca. Canned vegetables.
Animal Protein	Sugar Detox: Organic chicken, fish or turkey	Factory-farmed meats including: pork, beef, veal, sausage, cold cuts, canned meats, hot dogs
Grains & Beans	Vegan Detox: Non-gluten grains like quinoa and all beans	Gluten grains: wheat, barley, rye, couscous. Oats and soybean by-products.
Nuts & Seeds	Raw unsalted/unsweetened: almonds, cashews, walnuts, hazelnuts, brazil nuts, sesame seeds, pumpkin seeds	Peanut products
Dairy & Dairy Substitutes	Almond milk, rice milk, hemp milk, coconut milk	Cows milk, soy milk, non-dairy creamers, all cheese, cream cheese, cottage cheese, butter, yogurt (all types)
Sweeteners	None, except those in small quantities already listed in a recipe	Stevia, Xylitol, beet sugar, white and brown sugars, raw honey, 100% maple syrup, black strap molasses
Beverages	Green or herbal teas (non-caffeinated), water, fresh (juiced at home) vegetable juices	Commercial fruit juices, energy drinks, alcohol, caffeinated beverages, coffee, soft drinks
Oils & Vinegars	Extra virgin olive oil, coconut oil	Canola, sunflower and corn oil. Margarine, shortening and butter.
Herbs & Condiments	Vinegar: Apple cider, white wine, red wine, balsamic, rice vinegar. All fresh herbs and spices, mustard.	Commercial salad dressings, ketchup, relish, chutney, BBQ sauce, mayonnaise
Other	Small amounts of cocoa nibs, unsweetened cocoa powder	Candy, chocolate, energy bars, protein bars

Let's Talk About Fruits!

We love them! While fruits are filled with vitamins, minerals and fiber, having them in excess also means loads of added sugar. During Operation Cleanse, you eliminate all fruits except those in your daily smoothies. Keep your serving of daily fruits to about 1-1 ½ cup per day. Half a cup of fruit is the amount you can hold in one cupped hand.

Note: You get your fruit servings in your smoothies. That means no fruit snacks during the day!

GET YOUR GREENS ON

Do we need to remind you to eat your greens? Think of this as a pleasant reminder because greens, especially the dark, leafy ones, are loaded with vitamins and phytonutrients. Greens are plant nutrition power-players that will boost your immunity, reduce inflammation, balance your body, support heart health and your nervous system, strengthen bones, help with elimination, and give you gorgeous, glowing skin. They also increase your energy, and boost your mood.

Here are some ways you can incorporate more greens into your everyday cleanse routine as you think about how to prepare for Operation Cleanse.

HAVE A PLATE WITH 50% GREENS TWICE A DAY, LUNCH & DINNER

Unless you're drinking green smoothies 3 times a day, this is a fantastic habit to get into that'll keep your digestion operating at full capacity (remember greens = fiber = good bowel movements). Make it delicious with some homemade dressing (always opt for making your own dressing).

BLEND A GREEN POWER SMOOTHIE!

By the time we are done with Operation Cleanse, you will have an arsenal of recipes. Ever so often, add more greens and eliminate 1/2 of the fruits. The greener it is, the more punch you pack.

ENJOY A GREEN JUICE TOO!

Pressed green juices are available almost everywhere now and are a fantastic drink. If you are on the go, you can opt for pressed juices. We do not suggest making a habit out of them because they do not pack all the fiber you need for healthy digestion!

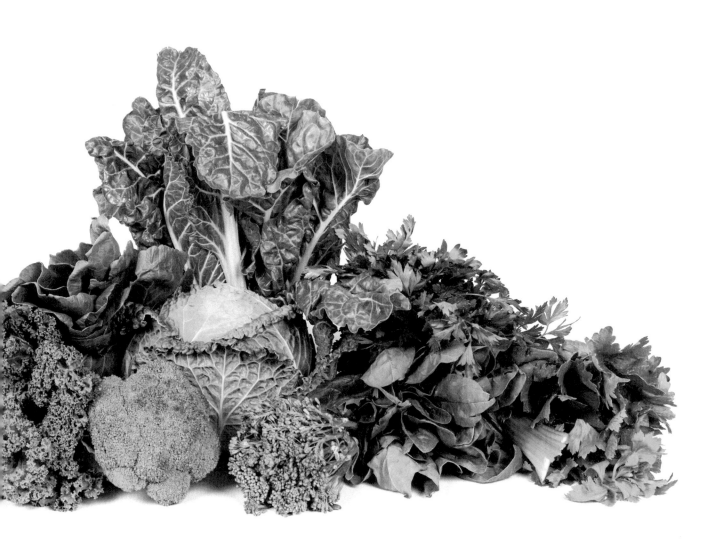

THE GREEN "YES" LIST

You can pick any of the veggies listed below and add them to any recipe to add more bulk or pack more nutrients. If there is a veggie you've never tried on here, now is your chance to try it!

HAVE AS MANY OF THESE AS YOUR HEART DESIRES

- Artichoke
- Arugula
- Asparagus
- Bean sprouts
- Bok choy
- Broccoli
- Brussels sprouts
- Cabbage
- Carrots
- Cauliflower
- Celery
- Chayote
- Chives
- Collard greens
- Cucumber
- Dandelion greens
- Eggplant
- Green beans
- Kale
- Leeks
- Mushrooms
- Okra
- Onions
- Parsley
- Peppers (red, green, yellow)
- Salad greens (all)
- Snap peas & Snow peas
- Squash (summer, spaghetti, zucchini)
- Swiss chard

here's a *tip!*

When in doubt, batch roast!

We can't stress enough how much we love batch roasting. It saves time and gives you the flexibility to add a bit of your roast to all your dishes.

Batch roast like a pro in 8 simple steps!

1. Peel and chop your veggies into bite sized portions
2. Set your oven to 350°F
3. Lightly spray your vegetables with extra virgin olive oil
4. Pick your fresh seasonings. Here are some combinations.
   - Salt, Pepper, Mashed Garlic
   - Cumin, Salt, Turmeric
   - Garlic, Fresh Lemon, Thyme
   - Rosemary, Peppercorn, Garlic
   - Thyme, Rosemary, Vinegar, Salt, Pepper
5. Evenly coat all vegetables with seasoning mix
6. Spread evenly in baking pan
7. Roast for 30-45 minutes until cooked through and browning
8. Enjoy on it's own, or add to other recipes of your choosing

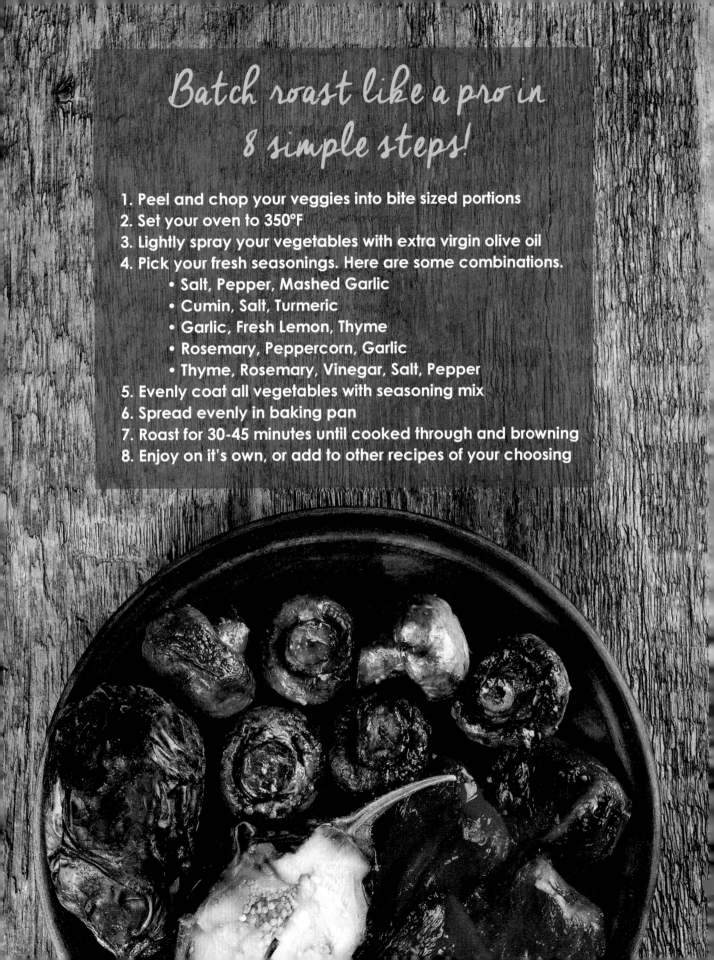

Blending 101

HOW TO STORE YOUR SMOOTHIES

You're busy, we know! Preparation is key when it comes to Operation Cleanse success. Some people say that storing your smoothies for 2 or 3 days means you do not get all the nutrients, that's false! We encourage you to prepare your smoothies ahead of time. As long as you store your smoothies in an airtight container (like mason jars) the freshness and nutrients will be there when you drink them. Just don't overdo it. Prepare them a maximum of three days in advance.

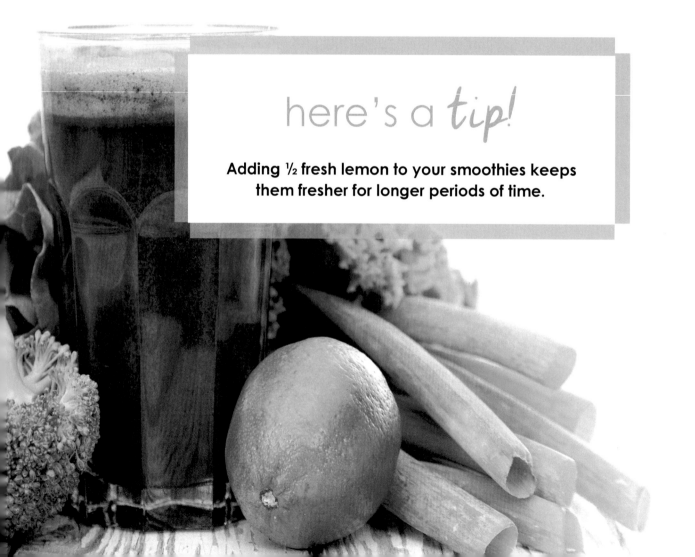

here's a *tip!*

Adding ½ fresh lemon to your smoothies keeps them fresher for longer periods of time.

MASTER SMOOTHIE RECIPE

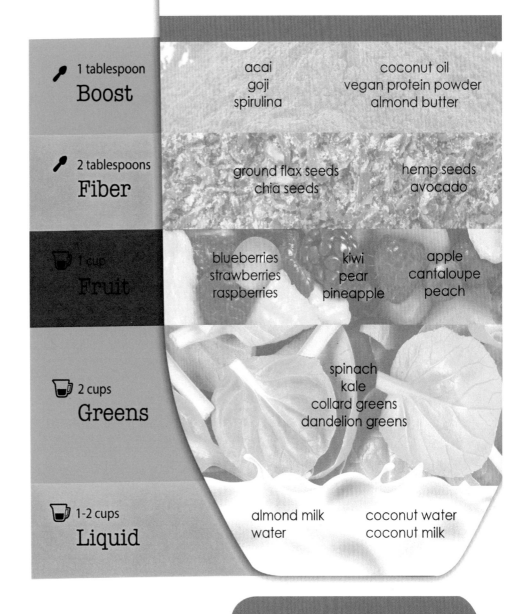

1 tablespoon **Boost**	acai, goji, spirulina — coconut oil, vegan protein powder, almond butter
2 tablespoons **Fiber**	ground flax seeds, chia seeds — hemp seeds, avocado
1 cup **Fruit**	blueberries, strawberries, raspberries — kiwi, pear, pineapple — apple, cantaloupe, peach
2 cups **Greens**	spinach, kale, collard greens, dandelion greens
1-2 cups **Liquid**	almond milk, water — coconut water, coconut milk

let's break it down...

CREATE YOUR SMOOTHIE

Green smoothies may possibly be one of God's best gifts. We love them and have included 24 of our favorites in the smoothie section in part 2. It's possible that you'll want to explore your own recipes and we know how easy it is to get lost in the thousands, possibly millions, of smoothie recipes out there. Here's the one smoothie recipe you need to keep in mind for the rest of your life.

here's a *tip!*

Always introduce your smoothie ingredients into your blender in order from lightest in weight to heaviest.

STEP 1: LIQUID

Depending on your desired thickness, add 1 ½ - 2 cups of liquid. We love drinking with a straw so we lean towards 2 cups. You can use anything from purified water to unsweetened almond milk. Coconut water is a great liquid base for any of the smoothies and adds additional sweetness when using bitter greens.

STEP 2: GREENS

Always add 2-3 large handfuls (or 2-3 cups) of leafy greens in your smoothies. Some of our favorites are kale and dandelion greens. If you are a newcomer to smoothies, go with baby spinach. Once you get into the smoothie lifestyle, add leafy herbs like cilantro, parsley and mint! Usually, we take a look at what is on sale and if it's leafy and green, we blend it!

STEP 3: FRUIT

It's easy to overdo it here! Remember, even fruits can mean too much sugar (even though it's natural sugar) and too much sugar, of any kind, means inflammation and imbalanced blood sugar. To avoid this, stick to ½ - 1 cup of fruit per smoothie. You can definitely mix and match the fruits but stick to ½ - 1 cup total.

STEP 4: FIBER

The greens and fruits in your smoothies have fiber, but it's never enough! Remember men need 38 grams and women need 25 grams of fiber daily in order to keep their digestion going. Add 2 tablespoons of your choice of chia seeds or ground flax seeds to all your smoothies to help you reach these targets.

STEP 5: BOOST IT

This is optional but highly recommended. If you are already committed to having your daily smoothies, why not add some extra benefits in the form of superfoods. Hemp and maca powder are two of our favorites (start with 1 tablespoon and increase from there).

STEP 6: TOP IT

Give your smoothie an additional kick with fresh herbs.

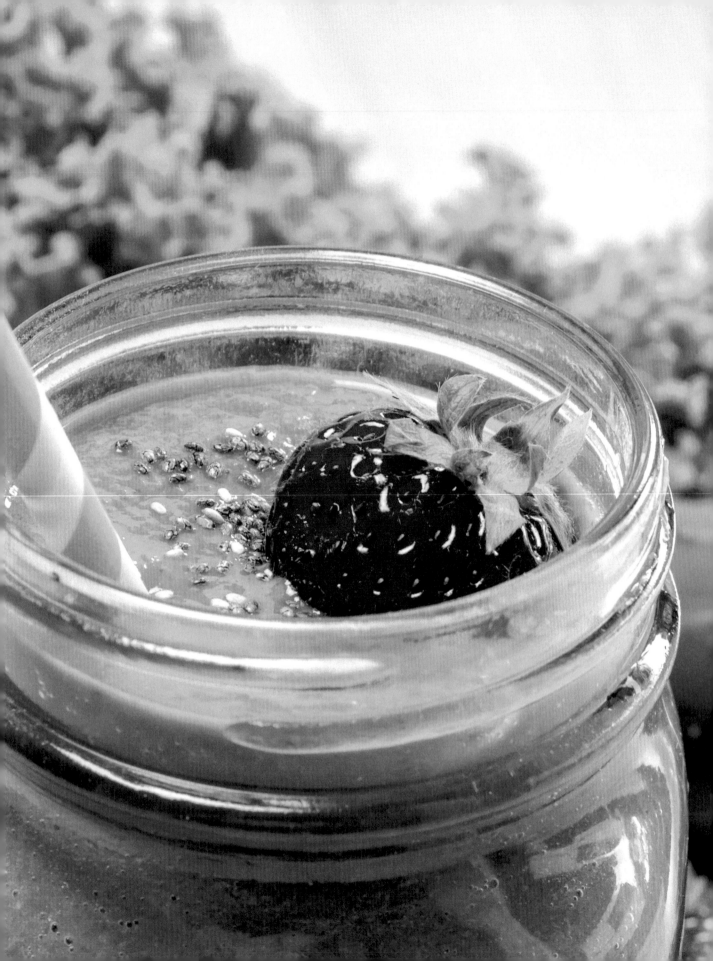

GIVE YOUR SMOOTHIES A BOOST!

Your body is nutrient dependent. It NEEDS food to function, and even to detox so your smoothies should always contain lots of greens, just enough fruits, fiber and protein. To turn your smoothies into super smoothies, let's superfood them up!

Superfoods are basically nutrient powerhouses that pack large doses of antioxidants, vitamins, and minerals in a small serving. They come in powder form, but also come in actual food form. For smoothie purposes, here are some of our favorite superfood powders and why you need to add 1 tablespoon to your next green smoothie!

MACA

The people of Peru have consumed maca for centuries for its energy-enhancing and mood-stabilizing capabilities. Traditionally, maca has also been used to regulate, support, and balance hormones. I'm talking about superfood capabilities like relieving cramps, hot flashes, and mood swings. Need another reason to add a tablespoon or two to your smoothie? Maca also helps improve collagen synthesis - that means supple, firmer and radiant skin!

GOJI

Goji berries have gotten their fame over the past few years with claims of helping to treat diabetes, hypertension, fever and even cancer. This immune boosting superfood contains more Vitamin C than oranges and more beta-carotene than carrots. For you, that means amazing skin and enhanced eye sight. When adding a tablespoon to your smoothie expect to add sweetness, it is after all a berry.

ACAI

If you have stepped inside a health food store in the recent past, you are bound to have seen acai everything! Acai is a super antioxidant which means they help with premature aging by keeping your cells renewed. They also have a nice amount of healthy fat and fiber to help promote cardiovascular and digestive health.

HEMP

If you are looking for a complete superfood to start off slow, hemp should top your list. Hemp is high in essential fatty acids and omega-3s, which can help fight heart disease and cancer. They are also a great source of added protein (to help keep you full) and a have a high Vitamin E content to help keep your immune system doing its thing! You can add hemp powder or hemp seed hearts to your smoothie – the benefits remain the same.

SPIRULINA

Gram for gram, this superfood has more protein than a steak without the artery clogging cholesterol that comes from most red meat sources. That means, spirulina can help keep you just as full as that steak can. Spirulina also contains its fair share of B vitamins which help give you an immediate energy boost. If you can get past the fishy smell (it's an algae), you are in for a detoxing treat. It's also packed with chlorophyll to help clear your blood of toxins and increase your oxygen levels.

COCONUT OIL

Coconut oil is considered the healthiest oil on earth. It helps protect against heart disease by increasing your good cholesterol, helps slow down the release of sugar into your bloodstream and helps to boost your metabolism. Adding a tablespoon to your smoothie can also help with your digestion if you are one to have a hard time going.

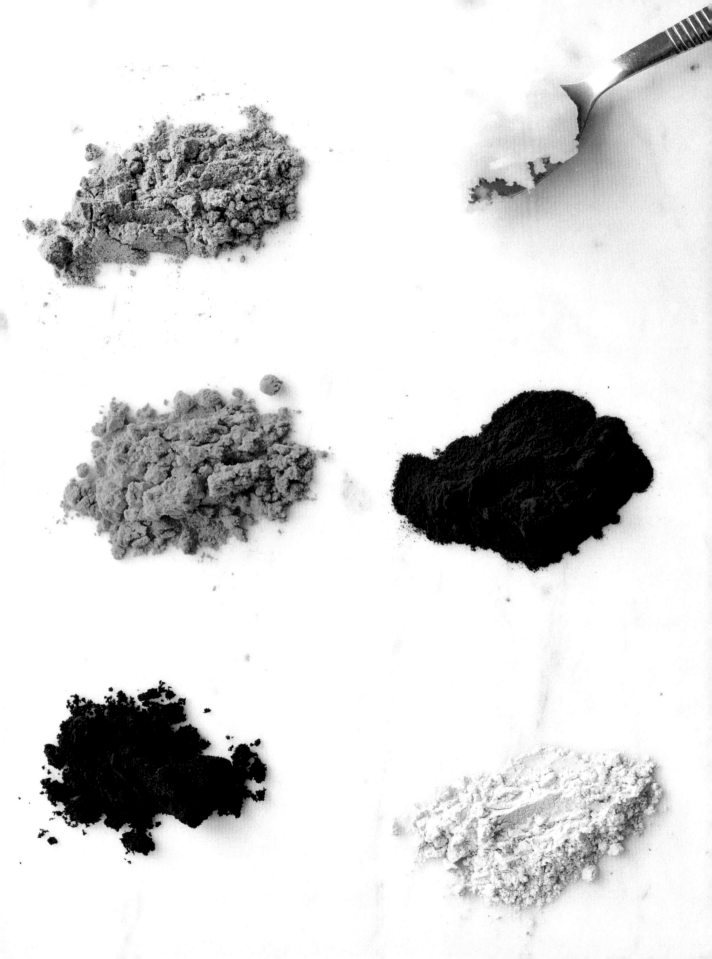

GOING ORGANIC

Most of the toxins found in our food come from pesticide residue. A surprising three fourths of 6,953 produce samples tested by the U.S. Department of Agriculture in 2014 contained pesticide residues. We know that for many, shopping 100% organic can be out of reach due to pricing, so we encourage you to focus your organic shopping to those fruits and vegetables that contain the most pesticides by using the the Dirty Dozen™ and Clean Fifteen™ lists. The Dirty Dozen™ is a list of produce that contains the highest levels of pesticides. If you eat fruits and vegetables from this list often, purchase organic as often as possible. The Clean Fifteen™ is a list of produce with the lowest levels of pesticides. Produce on this list doesn't necessarily need to be purchased organic. Both lists are arranged in order of pesticide content from highest to lowest.

DIRTY DOZEN™	CLEAN FIFTEEN™
Strawberries	Avocados
Nectarines	Sweet Corn
Peaches	Pineapples
Celery	Cabbage
Grapes	Sweet Peas
Cherries	Onions
Spinach	Asparagus
Tomatoes	Mangoes
Sweet Bell Peppers	Papayas
Cherry Tomatoes	Kiwi
Cucumbers	Eggplant
Hot Peppers	Honeydew Melon
Kale/Collard Greens	Grapefruit
	Cantaloupe
	Cauliflower

Source: EWG's 2016 Shopper's Guide to Pesticides in Produce™ and Environmental Working Group

Getting Your Kitchen Ready

Have you ever spent hours preparing for a party, special event, or vacation? Now, have you ever spent that much time planning your health? If the answer is no, here is your chance to change that habit. Having a successful cleanse takes time and preparation both mentally and physically.

YOUR KITCHEN ESSENTIALS

Prepare your kitchen with some of these basic tools.

MANDOLIN SLICER OR A SPIRALIZER

This kitchen gadget makes chopping so much easier. You need this to make "zoodles". If you don't know what zoodles are, get ready to have your mind blown! You can get a mandolin slicer or spiralizer on Amazon or in Bed Bath & Beyond for as little as $15. We've linked some of our favorites in the Shop section of OperationCleanse.com.

BLENDER

Need we say more? Nutri-Bullet, Magic Bullet, Vitamix or whatever you have at home will work. We highly recommend investing in a good blender. You will use it for smoothies, soups and dips during and after Operation Cleanse.

AIRTIGHT STORAGE CONTAINERS

Using airtight storage containers helps keep your food fresher longer vs. regular containers. You can find links for our favorites right on our website, OperationCleanse.com. During the cleanse, we encourage advance prepping so that you have NO EXCUSE to eat anything that you did not cook. Remember the golden rule of Operation Cleanse: if you don't make it, you don't eat it!

MASON JARS

We can't stress enough how awesome these are. You can store your smoothies, salads and soups in these for days with no worries. They are made of glass, helping you reduce chemical exposure from plastic. Amazon has them in bulk. We recommend the 'quart size, wide-mouth lid' option. Wide-mouth is easier to clean. At minimum, have 4 of these on hand.

FOOD PROCESSOR

Many of you probably have one collecting dust somewhere. The time for this baby to shine has come! This will make a great tool for dips, snacks and just overall chopping.

PANTRY ESSENTIALS

The following is a list of kitchen basics that you should have when preparing for Operation Cleanse. Check your pantry, you may already have many of these. Most of these basic ingredients will appear in your recipes so plan on having them.

- ☐ Extra virgin olive oil
- ☐ Coconut oil
- ☐ Almond butter
- ☐ Chia seeds
- ☐ Ground flax seeds
- ☐ Tahini
- ☐ Unsweetened almond milk
- ☐ Apple cider vinegar
- ☐ Balsamic vinegar
- ☐ Tamari Sauce or liquid aminos
- ☐ Sea salt
- ☐ Black pepper
- ☐ Fresh herbs like mint, cilantro and parsley

Anti-inflammatory and detoxifying herbs & spices like:
- ☐ Turmeric
- ☐ Cayenne pepper
- ☐ Chilli powder (or chilli flakes)
- ☐ Cumin
- ☐ Oregano
- ☐ Cinnamon
- ☐ Paprika

Pre-Cleansing

Four days before you decide to officially start your cleanse, take time to prepare. Over the past three years, we've had the pleasure of leading thousands on Operation Cleanse regimens, and the feedback has always been the same - those who plan ahead and properly pre-cleanse have an immensely better experience.   During your Pre-Cleanse, it's important to create an environment that will automatically guide you to the right choices during the two weeks. Setting up your mind, body, kitchen, work and overall schedule is essential for long-term health and Operation Cleanse success.

1. DETOX YOUR KITCHEN

Make today the last day your kitchen is under the reigns of the food industry! Get rid of:
- Anything that is not real food (aka packaged food)
- Any food or drink that contains sugar (including honey, molasses and agave) especially fruit juices.
- Any and all dairy items (including all types of yogurt and cheese)
- Any food with artificial sweeteners – basically anything with a food label

2. TAPER OFF CAFFEINE, DAIRY, ALCOHOL & SUGAR

This might be the most crucial Pre-Cleanse step to avoid major detox symptoms. If you drink caffeine (including caffeinated tea), today is the day to start tapering off. Reduce your intake by 1/4 then 1/4 of that then 1/4 of that. Make sure that by day 1 of Operation Cleanse you are at 0% of these toxins. We suggest you go cold turkey on sugar and alcohol three days before you officially start. Don't taper, just stop. If you pull the bandage slowly off these toxins, they hurt way more. On day 1 of your cleanse, you go full blown into eliminating all processed foods so it's better to start with the obvious ones first (like that chocolate cake!).

3. ALIGN YOUR MIND AND INTENTIONS

A revolution in the body, starts in the mind. Set aside some time to think and write down your intentions. The key is to write it because when you write you hold yourself more accountable. Here are some guiding questions:
- Why am I detoxing?
- What are my goals during Operation Cleanse?
- What are the top three things that stop me from living my best and healthiest life?
- What is my relationship with food?
- How will my life change once I learn what foods are my poisons?
- How can my life be different once I create vibrant health?

4. TAKE YOUR MEASUREMENTS

If your goal is weight loss, this is a must! Don't only look at the scale, put on those jeans that fit extra tight. Inflammation plays a huge role in the reason those pants don't fit. If your goal is to feel better, have more energy or vibrant looking skin – take before and after pictures! Pay close attention to your energy levels, and complexion, we are sure they will improve.

5. CREATE ACCOUNTABILITY

The research is endless that proves once you create accountability, you are more likely to achieve your goals. The social media age makes this so much easier! If you are social, we ask that you post your experience, let us see how you detoxed your kitchen, let us see the recipes you create, interact with us, share your experience with your friends and encourage them to join you. You can always find us using #OperationCleanse.

The Daily Cleanse Routine

After you Pre-Cleanse, you are ready to get into the real deal of Operation Cleanse. It's crucial that you get into a routine. Wake up at the same time each day. The goal is to eat every three hours so that you never get hungry. And if you happen to get hungry, eat! Remember, this is not about depravation. You can eat, as long as it is from your approved list. Your daily routine is broken up into 6 parts.

1. **When you wake up**, the first thing you should do is have a glass of room temperature water with the juice from half a lemon. Having lemon water in the morning is a habit we recommend you adopt post cleanse also. Lemon water boosts your immune system, aids digestion and cleansing, helps you lose weight, and reduces inflammation.

2. **A half hour after** your lemon water, you are ready for your morning smoothie. Pick a recipe from the smoothie section and go crazy! Be sure to drink slowly, there should be no rush here.

3. **2-3 hours after** your morning smoothie, you are ready for a mid-morning snack. Your mid-morning snack consists of nuts of your choice. Remember to get them unsalted and unsweetened. A serving is whatever fits in your hand.

4. Lunchtime! Aim to have lunch about **2-3 hours after** you have your nut mix. Pick any of the recipes in Part 2 based on the week you are in. Remember, there is no calorie counting. Eat as much as your heart desires.

5. **3 hours after** lunch its time to snack! Pick a snack recipe, your choice of veggie and dip away!

6. Your last meal should be **3-5 hours before you go to bed**. If you are looking to push weight loss, replace your meal with a smoothie. If you want to maintain weight, pick another recipe from the correct week and enjoy!

FILL IN YOUR EATING SCHEDULE BASED ON WHEN YOU WAKE UP

_____:_____ AM Wake Up: Drink 1 cup of water with ½ lemon

_____:_____ AM Breakfast: Daily smoothie

_____:_____ AM Mid-morning Snack: Handful of nuts

_____:_____ PM Lunch: Pick from recipes

_____:_____ PM Mid-afternoon Snack: Pick from recipes

_____:_____ PM Dinner: Pick from recipes or have a smoothie

the *12 hour* rule

We are sure you've heard, "don't eat after 7PM". While the idea is correct, you should understand why. It's important to give your digestive system a break from all the work it did during the day digesting the food you ate. To do this, we recommend you give yourself a break of 12 hours in between dinner and breakfast. Think about your wake up time and don't eat solids 12 hours before you plan to wake up.

Supplements

Over the years we've had the opportunity to work with many supplement companies. None has exceeded the quality and efficacy of Nature's Sunshine Products. It's also the only supplement company to be listed on the Forbes Most Trustworthy Companies list. You can shop all of these amazing products right on OperationCleanse.com

ESSENTIAL SUPPLEMENTS FOR OPERATION CLEANSE

The following is a list of herbal supplements to help boost your results and control your symptoms while cleansing.

MILD LAXATIVE

Like most Operation Cleanse participants, you're coming in from a diet high in refined carbs and animal protein and low in vegetables and whole grains. This means your bowel movements are less than optimal. As you begin adding Operation Cleanse approved foods into your diet, it's important to help the 'old stuff' move out. The more bowel movements you have while cleansing, the faster your detox symptoms start to disappear.

Introducing a gentle, herbal formula like the Nature's Sunshine CleanStart to your detox routine will ensure that your bowel movements remain abundant while cleansing.

VEGAN-BASED PROTEIN POWDER

Regardless of your reason for cleansing, dietary protein intake is essential to maintaining muscle mass and a strong body. Think of muscles as the furnace that fuels the rest of your body with energy. Once you start to lose muscle mass, we start to get flabby. We still haven't met the first person who wanted a flabby body!

Our clients love the Nature's Sunshine Love and Peas protein powder so much that they continue to use it post Operation Cleanse.

MAGNESIUM

Magnesium helps you relax, everywhere. It helps you fall asleep, and balances the nervous system. It can also help ease occasional constipation, and release tense, aching muscles. Magnesium also relieves headaches and migraines by relaxing your blood vessels.

You can drink Magnesium in capsule form or as a powdered drink – we love the one called Calm. You can also get a high dose of Magnesium in Epsom Salt baths during a warm 20-minute bath.

FOOD ENZYMES

Our bodies naturally produce enzymes to help break down our food to its smallest parts. Only when we completely digest our food can our cells utilize their nutrients. If your current diet high is high in processed foods, then your body is not accustomed to the work of breaking down whole foods.

Adding a digestion booster like the Nature's Sunshine Proactazyme helps your body take full advantage of the nutrition coming from your new, cleaner, whole food diet.

PROBIOTIC

Our gut is the home to billions of good and bad bacteria involved in an array of functions including boosting immunity and producing serotonin a.k.a. our happy hormone. Adding a multi-spectrum probiotic like Nature's Sunshine Probiotic Eleven to your routine floods your gut with a wide variety of good bacteria to help shift the balance from bad to good inside your digestive tract.

OPERATION CLEANSE KITS
WITH YOUR DAILY ROUTINE

Purchase your cleanse kits on OperationCleanse.com.

YOUR ROUTINE WITH THE BASIC KIT

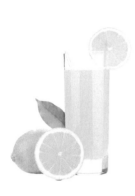
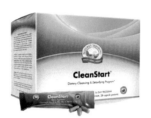
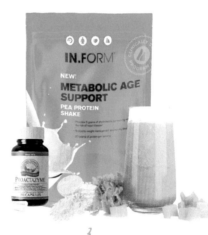
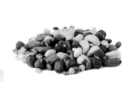

1
Cup of
water with
lemon

2
CleanStart
powder +
capsule packet

3
Morning smoothie +
enzyme capsules

4
Mid-Morning
snack

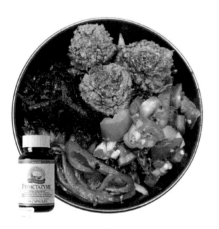

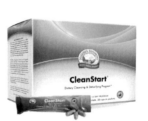
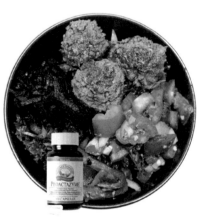

5
Lunch +
enzyme capsules

6
Mid-Afternoon
snack

7
CleanStart
powder +
capsule packet

8
Dinner +
enzyme capsules

YOUR ROUTINE WITH THE WEIGHT LOSS KIT

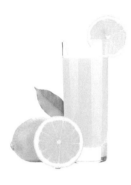

1

Cup of
water with
lemon

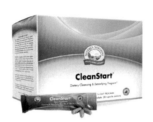

2

CleanStart
powder +
capsule packet

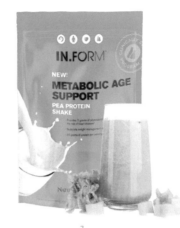

3

Morning smoothie

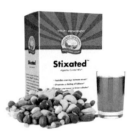

4

Stixated appetite
control mix +
snack

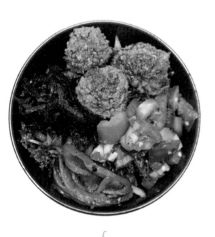

5

Lunch

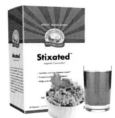

6

Stixated appetite
control mix +
snack

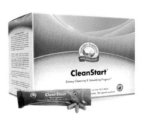

7

CleanStart
powder +
capsule packet

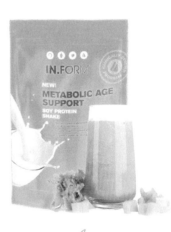

8

Dinner smoothie

Working Out & Eating Out

WHAT ABOUT WORKING OUT?

Did you know 80% of Americans do not get enough exercise according to the CDC (2015)? Movement helps your blood flow, improves your digestion and helps your brain to function. It even helps you sleep better (it's impossible to lose weight without good sleep), control your mood and balance your hormones.

We want to make sure that you are moving during Operation Cleanse. If you aren't a fan of the gym, this is the time to explore what may be getting in your way. Now is the time to shift your belief towards "I *can* find a physical activity that works for me." Keep it light. Remember, you are making a significant shift in your food so don't over exert yourself during the cleanse. Here are some of our favorite ways to get moving during a cleanse.

- Yoga
- Pilates
- Jogging
- Skip the elevator and take the stairs

Most of us just lack a little motivation. Here are some additional tips to motivate you.

BUDDY UP

There is endless research showing that people who are held accountable to others are more likely to stick with an exercise routine. Let's not forget peer pressure (of the good kind) is pretty effective. So find a friend you can exercise with and stick with it!

FIND YOUR REASON

Why do you want to get in shape? Is it to be a role model for your children? To live pain free? To fit in those jeans? To look good for your special someone? That's OK! Do whatever it takes and find whatever reason you need to get moving.

DO WHAT YOU ENJOY

The gym is not for everyone. Violet won't be caught dead near gym machines and you will never see Indhira on a track or treadmill. Violet loves Pilates and yoga, and Indhira loves a good kickboxing class. We have been able to find what works for us so we can stick with it.

BUY A NEW WORKOUT OUTFIT

This one is obvious! What's more motivating than a new outfit?

SET GOALS

This is possibly the most important. Set goals. How many times will you attend a class this week? How many miles will you run? Set those goals and hold yourself accountable to achieving them. S.M.A.R.T. goals work best. For example, I will power walk 1 mile, 2 days this week, at the park across the street before work. This goal is specific, measurable, achievable, realistic and time-based. Instead of I will workout this week.

EATING OUT

Sometimes, we just can't control the invitations to dine out whether it's birthdays, anniversaries or work related gatherings. There is no need to hide under a rock while cleansing, it's totally possible and completely OK to have dinner in a restaurant. Here's how to make it happen!

1. DON'T LEAVE YOUR HOUSE HUNGRY ... EVER

Before you leave your house, have some nuts, fruits, a quick smoothie or fresh juice. This will help you make better eating choices later in the evening.

2. HAVE A TALL GLASS OF LEMON WATER AS SOON AS YOU ARE SEATED

Drinking water will cut your hunger, rehydrate you after a long day, and give you some energy. It'll also fortify you to make good decisions, review the menu without going crazy, and allow you to calmly enjoy your company.

3. WINE OR NOT?
While cleansing, order sparking mineral water and lime or lemon. You've got this. After your cleanse; one is best, two is max.

4. SAY NO TO THE BREAD BASKET

You don't want to stare at those biscuits as they taunt you from the center of the table. Ask your waiter to please remove them. If your date is chowing down, nudge the basket across the table, out of arm's reach.

5. ORDER SALAD AS AN APPETIZER, ALWAYS

You can never overdose on raw greens, so take advantage of fresh greens while you're out. If they offer an option with a few nuts, or slices of pear, go for it. Order your vinaigrette on the side, and make sure that it's real olive oil and vinegar, or lemon.

6. LETS GO VEGAN!

Most restaurants have an assortment of fresh vegetables and you might be pleasantly surprised. Enjoy some brown rice, or quinoa if they have it. Only white rice? No thanks! Remember, your body will metabolize it as sugar almost instantly. You may as well have a cupcake! (not really, but you get the point).

7. SKIP DESSERT

You should be completely full and satisfied after this meal, so order an herbal tea to help you relax and ease your digestion.

When Things Get Rough

We've heard it and experienced it first hand. The first few days are HELL, but thankfully it's temporary and a sign that your body is detoxing! We call this a healing crisis (that's an actual term). It occurs when your body becomes overloaded by the toxins being released from within cells and tissues. When your cells purge toxins faster than they can leave leave the body, the temporary overload produces detox symptoms like the ones listed below.

Remember, they are temporary and should pass by day 4-5. It's a completely natural part of cleansing and one you must overcome to reach the other side.

These are the most common symptoms you can expect:
- headache
- skin eruptions (face and body)
- fever
- nausea
- bloating
- gas
- joint pains
- feeling mentally foggy
- unusual fatigue
- insomnia
- sleepiness
- congestion
- irritability
- muscle cramps
- aches and pains
- hot/cold flashes
- night sweats

Here are a few things we suggest when things get rough:

INFRARED SAUNA

Unless you've been living under a rock, you've heard of the long list of benefits from infrared saunas. Infrared light safely and deeply penetrates human tissue which get's the body sweating (a plus for detoxing), speeds up the metabolism (a plus, plus for weight loss), improves circulation and relaxes achy muscles.

HAVE A COLONIC

This is our favorite (seriously). Colonics or colon hydrotherapy, is a safe, effective method of removing waste from the colon by introducing filtered and temperature regulated water into the colon. End result? The waste is softened and loosened, resulting in evacuation through natural bowel movements.

GET A MASSAGE

Massages are not just for pampering. It's a therapeutic, healing modality that will keep you healthy, relaxed, and assist with cleansing too. Treat yourself to this luxury, soon.

GET A FACIAL

You may notice more acne or oily skin during your cleanse. This is your body using your skin to push out the toxins any way it can. A deep facial will help to cleanse and purify your skin much more than you can at home with over the counter washes or scrubs.

WHAT MORE CAN YOU DO

WATER

Drink plenty of water. Your body wants help eliminating the toxins that your cells are releasing. Flushing your bladder and intestines with pure water will make a big difference in your energy level during these 14 days. The guide we give clients on how much water to drink per day is at minimum half your body weight in ounces.

For those of you that can't stand the taste of water, infuse it with lemon, lime, mint or any fruits that you enjoy. An added bonus is that infusing your water helps to alkalize your body.

SLEEP

Give yourself a break! The first 48-72 hours is when most of the detox magic happens, but they will pass. Although most of us can function on less than the recommended 7-8 hours of sleep per night, we suggest that you do your best to get to bed early to ensure you get the full 7-8 hours during Operation Cleanse. Getting to bed and waking up at the same time also helps to regulate your sleep/wake cycle for life post Operation Cleanse.

here's a *tip!*

If at all possible, make room for a nap if you feel less than great the first couple of days. Have confidence that any fatigue you feel will pass.

here's another *tip!*

If weight loss is your goal, it's not possible to lose weight without enough sleep.

Ending Your Cleanse

PREPARE FOR DAY 15

Once you're coming into the home stretch, all your beautiful work will be for nothing if you drive off the cliff back into sugar, gluten, processed foods, dairy, and inflammation-land. Instead, think about what you enjoyed and will keep post cleanse, to keep you balanced, clear and energized.

Preparing for day 15 is essential for long lasting results. During Operation Cleanse, you left your crazy, busy life with it's constant demands and somehow you made time to shop for healthy foods, made yourself a smoothie, prepared a fresh salad, explored new foods, you even read the restaurant menu with a new and improved point of view. You've nurtured yourself. Congratulations!

Now, try to hold onto it on day 15, and the week after, and the week after that. Make self-care a habit and we promise that you will feel like your best self! Think about what you loved and what will be most meaningful for you to keep as a new lifestyle.

Here are some ways to help you prepare.

1. GO GROCERY SHOPPING

Carve out time over the weekend to shop for your week. Stock your cupboards with healthy treats. Fill your fridge with greens and fruits. Keep going!

2. KEEP UP WITH YOUR MORNING SMOOTHIE

Your morning shake (or smoothie), is a fantastic way to wake up and start your day. You will nurture this healthy habit during your cleanse. After your cleanse, incorporate superfoods and explore other recipes so you don't get bored.

3. TRY SOMETHING NEW

Which recipe did you NOT get to? Do you need to work on sugar cravings? Need more sleep? Review the past 14 days, and set some goals for the coming weeks. Visit OperationCleanse.com to see how we can help you one-on-one.

4. RAW FOODS

Raw food refers to any whole food that is uncooked and not heated to above 115°F. Foods in their natural, raw state contain live enzymes, and benefit your absorption of vital nutrients. Eating more raw foods leads to clarity, feeling more alive and energized, and gorgeous, glowing skin.

You will eat a lot of raw foods during Operation Cleanse, in smoothies, vegetable juices, and salads, so aim to keep a high percentage of raw foods in your daily menu after as well. A smoothie for breakfast, green juice as a snack, or a salad at lunch and dinner. If you have trouble digesting raw foods, incorporate a food enzyme. You can shop on OperationCleanse.com.

5. DIGESTIVE & GUT MAINTENANCE

Cleansing has helped to balance your gut by killing off yeast and bad bacteria. This is the perfect time to replace the bad bacteria with healthy ones. Adding a high quality probiotic to your daily regimen would a great start. You can always shop on OperationCleanse.com for our favorite probiotics.

If you find yourself "clogged" for just a single day, go ahead and overdose on green juices, flaxseed, chia seeds and plenty of water. Make sure you continue to maintain regular bowel movements.

6. CREATE YOUR OWN PERSONAL FOOD POLICY

This is the key to success when it comes to embracing a new lifestyle. We encourage you to go ahead and create a policy that works for you.

THE RE-INTRODUCTION

On day 15, you will have successfully removed several problematic foods from your daily diet and you will feel amazingly good. Then what? The Re-Introduction phase is the ultimate opportunity to test and see which of these foods is the culprit of your bloating, fatigue, skin conditions or constipation.

What foods are you intolerant to? By reintroducing foods one at a time after eliminating them for a two-week period you get to see first hand what you are sensitive or intolerant to. By "see" we mean almost immediate bloating, stomach cramps and the like after eating the offending food. Let's review how to add foods back in to test for food sensitivities or intolerances.

Take a look back at the "NO" List. We eliminated caffeine, alcohol, dairy, and gluten along with many processed foods. Was there a food you ate often prior to Operation Cleanse? That's where you should start. For example, if you ate cheese every day, eat a slice of cheese or two on day 1 or 2 post-Operation Cleanse. Have it just once and be sure to eat high enough quantities in order to get a reaction. For example, a whole tomato, 2 eggs, a glass of milk, or a few ounces of cheese, 2 slices of bread, and so on. Do not reintroduce any other foods the day you eat cheese. This way you're not left wondering which of the foods made you feel crappy.

Here we listed a sample re-introduction schedule and common reactions. This is not a complete list of reactions but should be enough for you to get an idea of what to look for.

DAY 1

Add dairy. Common reactions are stomach pains, gas, bloating, headaches, mucus, stuffy nose, nasal drip, and intestinal issues.
Wait 2 days.

DAY 3

Add gluten like bread or wheat pasta. Common reactions are stomach pain, intestinal issues, and diarrhea.
Wait 2 days.

DAY 5

Add a processed meat like a sausage. Common reactions include abdominal pain,diahhrea, cramping or joint pain.
Wait 2 days.

DAY 7

Add sugar and desserts. Common reactions are stomach pain, hyper energy, brain fog, nausea.
Wait 2 days.

DAY 9

Add alcohol. Common reactions are bloating, swelling, headache (trust us, your tolerance is low. Take it easy).
Wait 2 days.

DAY 11

Add coffee. Common reactions are anxiety, anger, nervousness, and sleeplessness.

You may not need, or want to test for all of these.

For example, you may already know that alcohol is problematic, or that coffee gives you jitters and is highly addictive, and that refined/processed sugars from white rice and sweets is something that you should avoid anyway. Whatever you decide, test for dairy and gluten, since they are inflammatory for so many people, and likely played a role in your daily diet.

Take advantage of this time to get information that will help you move forward. Then act on it. If you do get a reaction, believe it, trust your body. It's not a fluke, or coincidental.

F.A.Q.

THE BASICS

We encourage you to wake up at least an hour before you need to leave your house. Many times we wake up in the morning in such a rush that we don't take 10 minutes to think about ourselves. We understand some of you have children and lead busy lives, but we encourage you to take some time in the morning, meditate and connect with your intentions for detoxing.

HOW DO I KNOW EXACTLY WHAT TO BUY?

Refer to the Getting Your Kitchen Ready in Part 1 to check for what you already have. These lists will help you understand what your kitchen should ALWAYS look like. Check what you're missing from the recipes that you choose for breakfast/lunch/dinner and shop as needed. Make sure you always go shopping with a list to avoid wasting time and temptations!

WHAT WILL I HAVE FOR LUNCH AND DINNER?

You need to take some time to look at the recipes and decide which you will prepare. Be sure to pick recipes that go with the appropriate week in the cleanse. Once you decide, purchase based on the ingredients in that recipe. We included the Pantry Essentials List so you are never missing the staples needed for a successful cleanse. You can use this list and combine it with the Green "Yes" List to make your own recipes.

If you come up with an amazing new recipe, share it with us using #OperationCleanse so that we can see the magic you create.

WHAT IF I DON'T HAVE TIME TO PREPARE FOODS EVERY DAY?

We encourage you to meal prep! On any given night with an hour or two, pick the foods you want to make, make them and pack them. You'll have food prepared for up to 3 days. Trust us, it makes the day and cleanse so much smoother. If you are on the go and find that you do not have time to prep, make sure you eat based on the "Yes" Lists. A safe restaurant option is always a salad (but this gets boring). Make sure you always skip the dressing and only use Balsamic Vinegar or Olive Oil and Vinegar. Also ensure that the salad is Dairy-Free.

WILL I BE HUNGRY?

No way! We actually have clients ask us, "I am always stuffed, how will I lose weight?!?!." These clients are pleasantly surprised that at the end of the cleanse, their weight and measurements go down. Remember, Operation Cleanse was created to show you how easy it can be to eat right and feel great. We want you to try all the recipes and find ways to make them your own using approved ingredients.

CAN I REPLACE INGREDIENTS?

There is a difference between not liking an ingredient and having an allergy. If you have a food allergy, of course use something else (as long as it is approved). We included a Food Substitution List in Part 3. If you simply do not like an ingredient just remember why you started Operation Cleanse. Your goal is to explore, so like we say to picky children: ***try it first, then decide***. Even when you hate it, remember your taste buds may require adapting. Try it twice before you decide you don't like it.

CAN I WORK OUT?

We certainly suggest that you work out LIGHTLY during Operation Cleanse. It's important that you release all the toxins you can and sweating is a great way to do so. We recommend yoga, pilates and light cardio.

I WANT TO GO OUT TO EAT! HOW CAN I DO THAT WITHOUT RUINING MY CLEANSE?

We understand – and it's fine to eat out. Just be prepared to exercise some serious willpower. Most places will have sides of vegetables or salads. And if not, talk to the restaurant and ask them what options they can offer you. Broth-based soups are generally another good choice (steer away from cream-based soups). You must 100% skip any alcohol (yes, wine also) and dessert. Good luck! In all honesty, we recommend skipping the outings while cleansing. Take a look at the Eating Out section in Part 1.

I'M STILL HUNGRY... CAN I EAT MORE THAN THE PLAN SAYS?

You need to listen to your body. If you're craving certain foods, you're often actually craving nutrients. Depending on the amount of activity you do, you may need more food than our meal plan suggests.

If so, fill the gap with snacks from the recipe section or more veggies from the Green "Yes" List. You may also need to eat a little more than a serving size (of veggies), and that's okay. Make sure you hydrate yourself with water, or herbal teas. Keep yourself busy and it'll soon be time for the next meal!

IS IT OK TO MAKE MY GREEN SMOOTHIES THE NIGHT BEFORE?

Yes, you can definitely blend your green smoothies the night before (even three days ahead of time). Just store them using mason jars with airtight lids to limit oxidation. If you plan on using chia seeds, add them in the morning, if not they will turn smoothies into a jelly if left to sit over several hours.

WHAT HAPPENS IF I BREAK THE GUIDELINES OF OPERATION CLEANSE?

Don't beat yourself up about it, but jump right back in. Think about what you struggled with and try to work on that area of weakness. We want you to get the most benefit from Operation Cleanse, so try to commit as much as you can.

WHAT IF I START TO FEEL SICK DURING OPERATION CLEANSE?

This is completely normal and it even has a name - Herxheimer Reaction aka Healing Crisis. As the body adjusts to the new healthier foods and tries to eliminate the toxins built up from your old lifestyle, it's more than possible to feel a headache, fatigue, irritable or like you're coming down with a cold at the start of Operation Cleanse. After a few days, you should start to feel great with a sense of well-being we can only describe as pure magic.

WILL THE SUPPLEMENTS I TAKE CAUSE SIDE EFFECTS?

The supplements we recommend with Operation Cleanse are proven effective and gentle for 99% of our clients over the past 10 years we have worked with this brand. If you are taking a prescription medication, check with your primary care physician before using any supplements. You can purchase all our supplements right on OperationCleanse.com.

I DON'T WANT TO LOOSE ANY WEIGHT, WHAT DO I DO?

If you do not want to lose weight while cleansing, simply go for a full meal for dinner instead of a smoothie and make your morning smoothie as large as a 32 oz. Regardless, you may feel your clothes fit a bit more loosely due to loss of inflammation.

HOW MANY CALORIES ARE IN THE OPERATION CLEANSE RECIPES?

We purposely leave out calories from the recipes because the LAST thing we want you to focus on is counting calories. Even though we've purposely left calories out, all the recipes have been nutritionally analyzed and balanced by Violet, so trust that you are getting all (and even more) nutrition than you normally would.

IS OPERATION CLEANSE SAFE IF I AM PREGNANT OR BREASTFEEDING?

While pregnant, we do not recommend taking any supplements or starting strict diet regimens unless your primary care physician OK's you doing so. While breastfeeding, Operation Cleanse recipes are balanced and completely healthy. The one exception while breastfeeding is that we suggest doing Operation Cleanse without supplements and eat as much as your heart desires from the approved lists.

CAN I DO IT WITH MY KIDS?

Many kids enjoy the smoothies and many of the recipes in Operation Cleanse and parents find that cooking for the entire family makes life easier. We encourage you to test recipes with your kids to get them on a path to healthier eating. When kids help in food preparation, they are more likely to eat the foods you make.

IF I HAVE A FOOD ALLERGY, WHAT DO I DO?

You know your body better than anyone else. If you come across a recipe with an ingredient you are sensitive or allergic to, don't just eliminate it, replace it with a different fruit, vegetable or nut of your choice. See the Food Substitution List in Part 3.

WHAT IF I HAVE INSULIN-DEPENDENT DIABETES OR ANOTHER CHRONIC DISEASE?

While we do use many of the Operation Cleanse recipes with ALL of the clients at our centers, My Wellness Solutions, we suggest checking with your primary care physician before embarking on any new diet regimen.

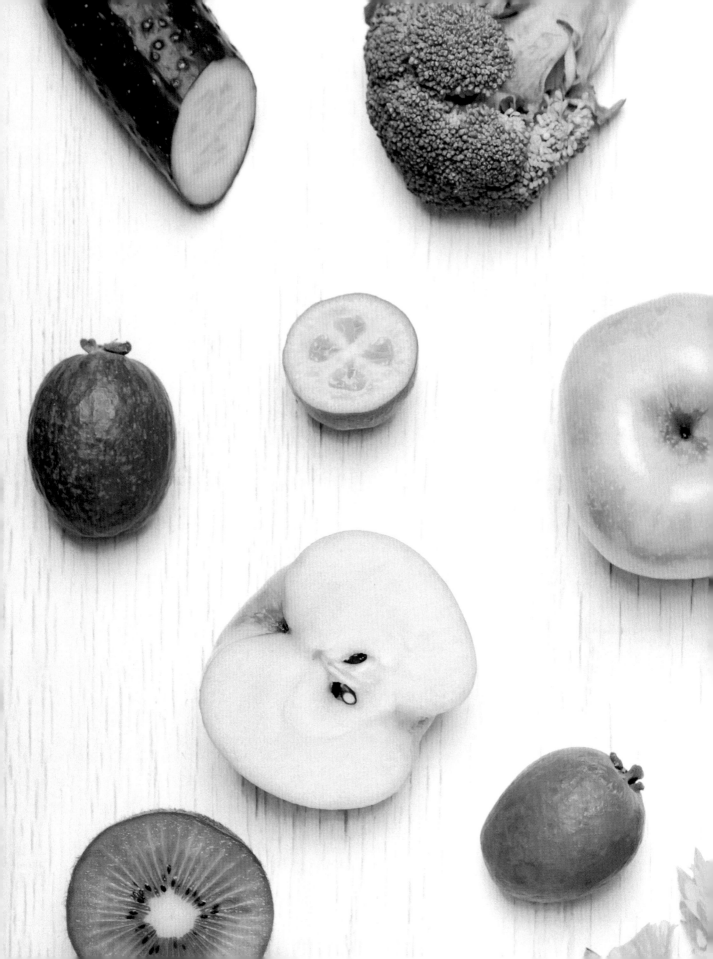

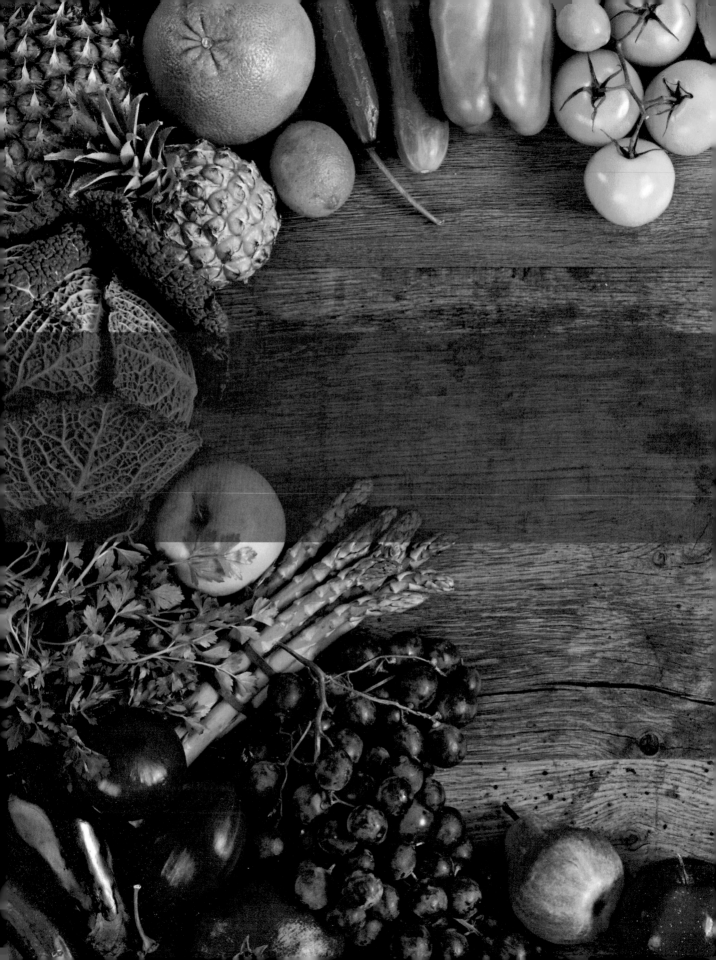

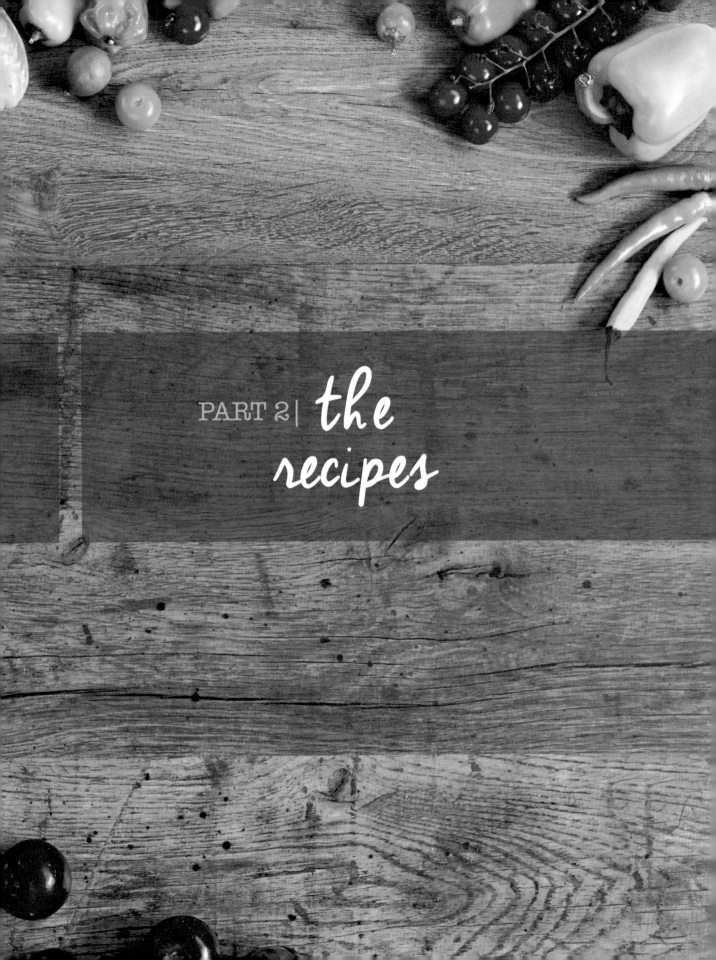

PART 2 | *the recipes*

Recipes with Endless Possibilities

Use approved ingredients, additional green vegetables, and get creative with the recipes. Just remember...

EAT WHAT YOU NEED

Most of the recipes in the book are suggested as 1 serving – but if you feel it's not enough, mix and match recipes or double up on one recipe. Soups for example tend to have less calories and protein which may leave you feeling hungry. If you have a soup, eat as much as you want until you are full or add a salad from the recipes to ensure you are full.

PERSONALIZE THE RECIPES

All recipes are simple to make and designed for you to combine or have alone with a side of vegetables from the Allowed List. This is the best part of Operation Cleanse. You can easily add lots of veggies, healthy fats, whole grains and starchy veggies (during Vegan Detox) to any meal and your choice of animal protein (during Sugar Detox). Get creative and have fun!

ADD YOUR CHOICE OF PROTEIN

Proteins are the building blocks of the body. Can you imagine a building without concrete or cement blocks? Without protein, your body would crumble. Most think of chicken, turkey, or another animal-source when we say protein, but there are countless plant-based sources of proteins to chose from including green leafy vegetables, beans and legumes, nuts and seeds, and even quinoa and oats.

During Sugar Detox feel free to have chicken, turkey or fish seasoned with any of the herbs and spices in the Allowed List. When we say turkey for example, we mean real turkey, not turkey cold cuts!

WHEN YOU WAKE UP

First thing in the morning, have a glass of room temperature water with ½ lemon. Having lemon in the morning helps to kick start your digestive system and metabolism. After this, follow the daily routine you created in Part 1.

SUPPORT YOURSELF

We're all about making sure you get enough nutrients each day. Our serving sizes are suggestions to start with. Figuring out how much is best for you to eat each day takes time and experimentation. If you exercise, eat more. Eat slowly and mindfully until you are about 80% full - satisfied, but not stuffed! Remember, calories do not matter when you are eating the right foods.

And finally...

Food should not only taste great, it's MUST make you FEEL great! If you're eating foods that make you feel like there's a brick in your stomach or you want to take a nap after, you may need to double check out what you're putting in that beautiful body.

THE OPERATION CLEANSE BOWL

The OC Bowl can easily be applied to ALL your meals during this cleanse. You will find that you may have leftovers for some recipes. Putting it all together in a bowl is the perfect way to save time in the kitchen! To create your own bowl, simply do the following:

- Select at least 1 ingredient from each category below
- Have the veggies raw, steamed, roasted, or sautéed
- When choosing a protein or carb, be sure the ingredient is allowed for the detox week you are in. Remember, no animal protein during Vegan Detox and no starchy vegetables or grains during Sugar Detox

GREENS	PROTEINS	FATS	VEGGIES	CARBS	ADD-ONS
Arugula	Beans	Avocado	Bell peppers	Butternut squash	Apple cider vinegar
Kale	Eggs	Nuts	Broccoli	Millet	Fresh herbs
Mustard greens	Nuts	Olive oil	Carrots	Quinoa	Home-made dressings
Romaine	Organic chicken or turkey	Olives	Cauliflower	Sweet potatoes	Nutritional yeast
Spinach	Seeds	Seeds	Cucumbers		
Swiss chard	Wild-caught fish	Sesame oil	Green beans		
		Truffle oil	Mixed veggies		
			Snap peas		
			Zucchini		
			Any veggies you love!		

put it all together!

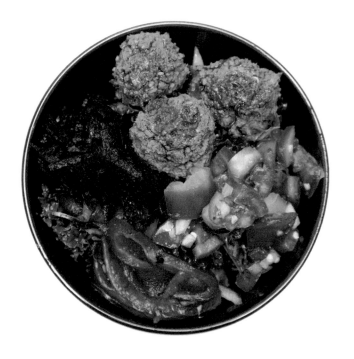

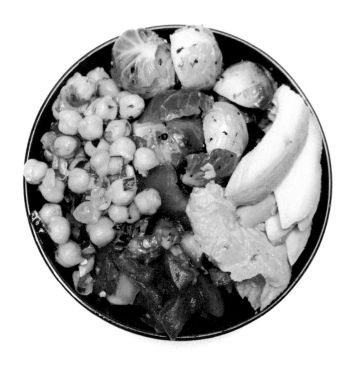

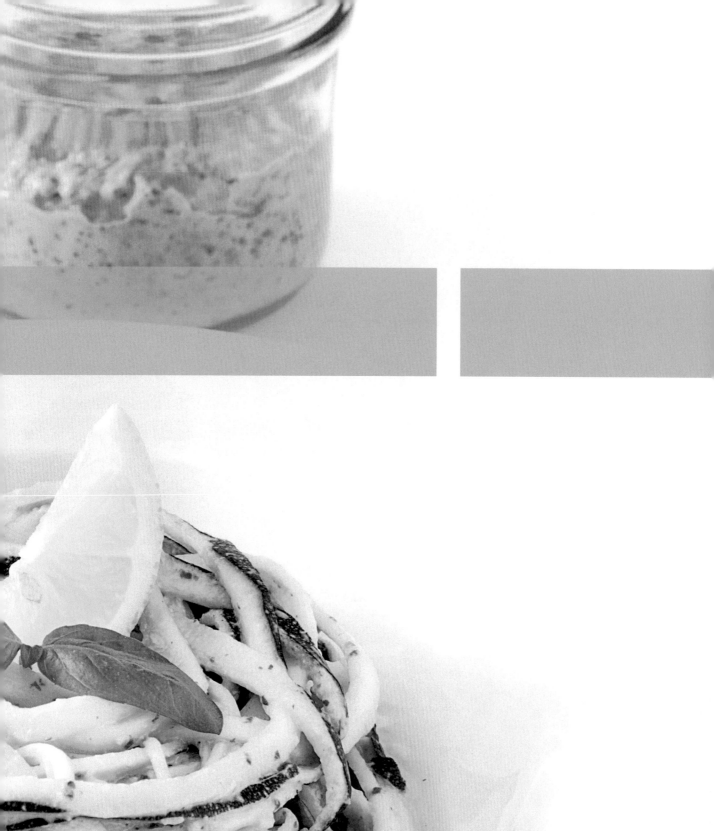

The Vegan Detox

LET'S GO VEGAN!

By eliminating animal protein of all kinds, we force you out of your comfort zone and target sources of excess bloating. This week it's all about discovering delicious quinoa recipes, root vegetables and beans in order to keep you full. Your goal this week is to perfect quinoa dishes. We hope that after you get it right, you never go back to white rice again!

CAULIFLOWER PIZZA CRUST

This recipe is all about the "crust" - it's made without any of the standard "dough" ingredients, no gluten, no dairy, no grains, nothing but goodness from cauliflower and some fun ingredients we want you to explore.

Keep in mind that this isn't your regular pizza crust, so expect a different texture. Since all ovens are different, the time to get to your desired texture may vary. The dough is very fragile after it's baked so be gentle! Even if it falls apart – it tastes great! Once you have the crust you desire, the topping possibilities are endless! You can bake it longer to have a "cracker" or you can top it with cold ingredients (think avocado toast with this crust!)

Ingredients
1 small head cauliflower, chopped
1 cup of water
2 whole eggs
3 tablespoons nutritional yeast
1 tablespoon coconut flour, or quinoa flour
1/2 teaspoon garlic powder
2 garlic cloves, minced
1 teaspoon sea salt, more to taste
1/2 teaspoon dried basil
1/2 teaspoon dried oregano
Fresh ground black pepper, to taste

Directions

1. Preheat oven to 450°F.

2. Lightly boil the cauliflower for 3-5 minutes or until slightly soft. Blend with 1 cup of water to smooth.

3. Place the cauliflower into a cheesecloth or paper towels over a large bowl and squeeze the excess water from the cauliflower.

4. Let the cauliflower sit for about 10 minutes, returning to squeeze any remaining water. Discard the liquid. The end result will resemble a puree.

5. Add remaining ingredients into the bowl and mix.

6. Spread "dough" about 1/2 inch thick into either 1 large pizza shape or 2 small pizza rounds on parchment paper. Avoid spreading the "dough" too thin as the moisture will cause it to crack and pull away from rest of the dough. We like leaving ours about 1/2 inch thick.

7. Bake at 450°F for about 20 minutes, until the top is golden brown and firm to the touch. Flip half way through the baking process to make sure both sides are cooked well to your liking.

8. Remove from oven and add toppings. Bake another 10-15 minutes until toppings are warmed and melted.

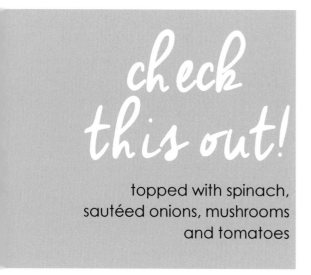

check this out!

topped with spinach, sautéed onions, mushrooms and tomatoes

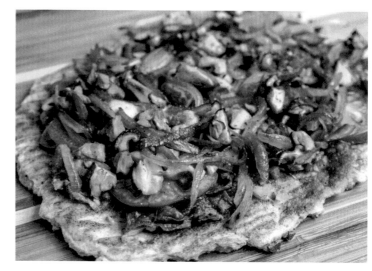

ROASTED POTATO SALAD WITH GREEN BEANS & SHALLOT DRESSING

Ingredients
6 small red potatoes, halved
1 sweet potato, cut into bite sized cubes
2 tablespoons extra virgin olive oil
Sea salt, to taste
1 cup green beans, trimmed and cut into 2 inch strips
4 shallots, finely sliced

Dressing
3/4 cups extra virgin olive oil
1/4 cup sherry vinegar
1/2 shallot, peeled and sliced, sautéed
3 tablespoons Dijon mustard
2 teaspoons sea salt, to taste

Directions
1. Preheat oven to 350°F.

2. Toss potatoes, olive oil, and salt in medium bowl. Transfer potatoes to parchment-lined sheet tray, and roast in oven until caramelized, stirring occasionally, approximately 40 minutes. Remove potatoes from oven and allow them to cool.

3. While potatoes are roasting sauté green beans and shallots. Salt to taste. Be sure not to overcook to avoid making them soggy.

4. Combine potatoes in medium bowl with green beans and shallots.

5. Blend dressing ingredients in blender until smooth. Add dressing to potatoes, to taste.

6. Serve over your choice of leafy greens or cooked quinoa.

CITRUS BEET SALAD

This iron packed salad is delicious on its own or can be added to a bed of dark leafy greens. Option to add Chickpea Meatballs for additional protein.

Ingredients
3 red beets, diced (option to use golden beets)
1 large segmented orange, peeled, chopped
1 tablespoon, extra virgin olive oil
1/2 cup hemp seeds
Fresh parsley to garnish
Sea salt, to taste

Directions
1. Preheat oven to 350°F.
2. Toss diced beets in olive oil. Salt to taste. Place on a baking sheet and roast until tender. Approximately 35-40 minutes.
3. Remove from oven to cool. When cooled, toss oranges and beets in a bowl. Lightly crush the oranges to release juices.
4. Top with hemp seeds and parsley. Serve over your choice of greens or quinoa.

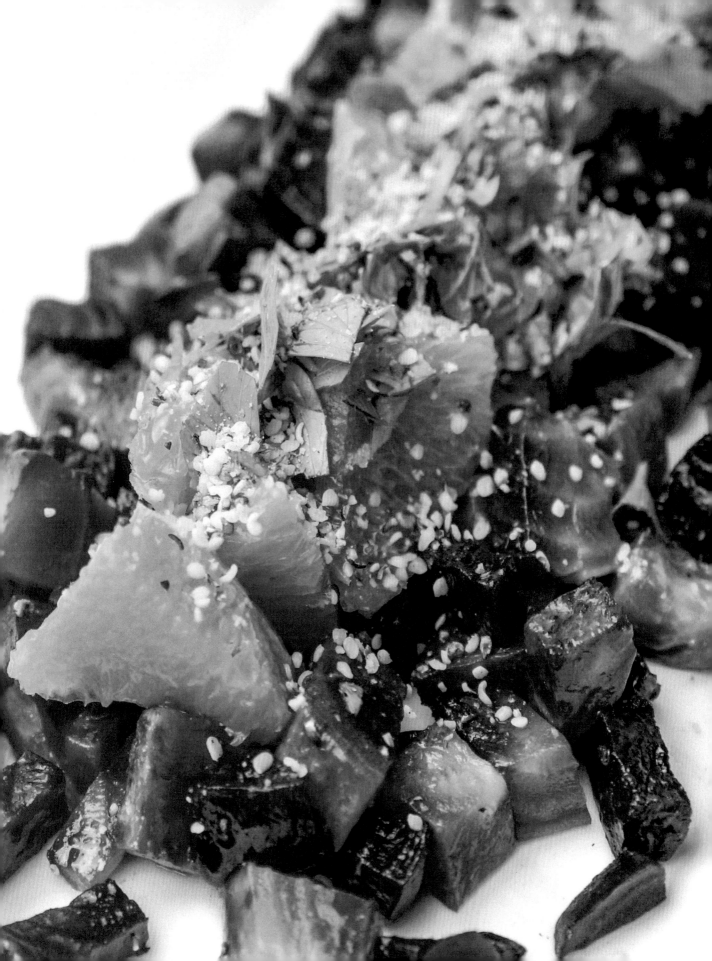

CHICKPEA MEATBALLS

This recipe is a must! We promise these "meatballs" are absolutely amazing. You can have 2-3 as a quick mid-afternoon snack, serve them over your choice of zoodles or add them to any salad. This recipe will make about 20-24 chickpea meatballs, your serving size is about 3-4 balls.

Ingredients
3 tablespoons extra virgin olive oil
4 garlic cloves, minced
1/4 cup sweet onion, chopped
1 egg, beaten
1 teaspoon tamari sauce, or more to taste
1/2 cup nutritional yeast
1/4 cup rolled oats
1/3 cup hemp seeds
1/2 cup walnuts, chopped
1/2 cup fresh basil, chopped
1/4 cup sun-dried tomatoes, chopped
1/2 teaspoon dried oregano
1/2 teaspoon sea salt, or more to taste
Pinch of red pepper flakes, to taste
Fresh ground black pepper, to taste
1 15-ounce can chickpeas, drained, rinsed and dried

Directions
1.   Preheat oven to 350°F.

2.   In a medium heated skillet, add 1 tablespoon olive oil and onions. Sauté for 2-4 minutes until they start to soften. Add garlic, a pinch of sea salt and black pepper. Cook 5 minutes until fragrant.

3.   In a food processor or blender, combine sauté with nutritional yeast, hemp seeds, egg, chopped walnuts, oats, basil, sun dried tomatoes, oregano, sea salt, black pepper, red pepper flakes, tamari sauce, remaining olive oil, and chickpeas. Pulse together until smooth. Add more olive oil as needed to soften the mixture.

4. Pour mixture into mixing bowl. Adjust seasonings to taste before you start rolling into balls. Use olive oil or water to coat your hands to prevent the meatballs from sticking to your hands as you roll your balls. Place on oiled baking sheet.

5. Bake until golden brown. Allow to cool before removing from baking sheet. Carefully handle if rotating or flipping the chickpea balls during the baking process.

ENDLESS POSSIBILITIES

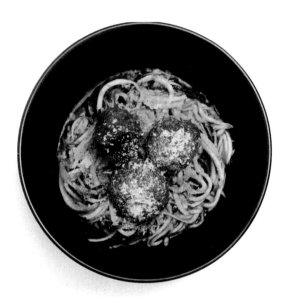

chickpea meatballs + tomato zoodles

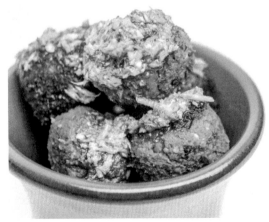

chickpea meatballs + chimichurri

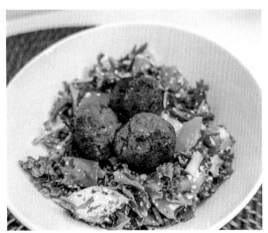

chickpea meatballs + kale

CAULIFLOWER AND ASPARAGUS SOUP

Ingredients

1 head cauliflower, roughly chopped
1 pound asparagus, cut to 1 inch pieces
6 cups low sodium vegetable stock
4 garlic cloves, minced
1 onion, chopped
Sea salt and pepper, to taste
Fresh herbs of your liking. Rosemary, thyme, and cayenne are recommended

Directions

1.   In medium pan add oil, garlic and onions. Sautee for 3 minutes.

2.   Add cauliflower, asparagus and fresh herbs. Toss for 4 minutes. Add broth and bring to boil until cooked.

3.   Remove and transfer to blender. Season with salt and pepper to taste.

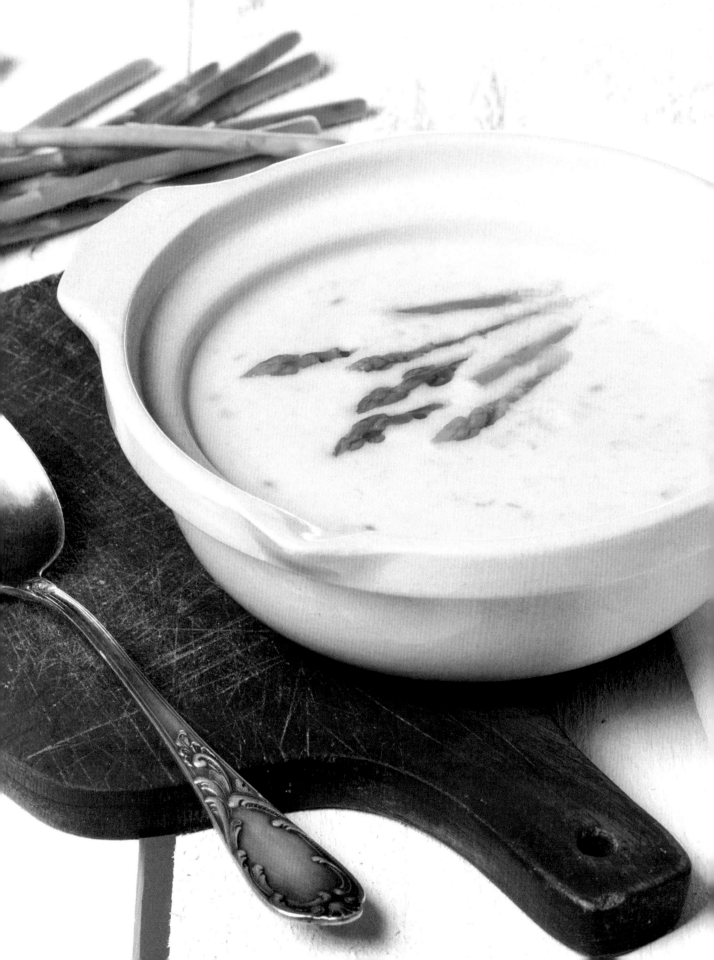

PERFECTING YOUR QUINOA

Quinoa (pronounced KEEN-wah) is a fluffy, high-protein seed that's loaded with iron, magnesium, and fiber. It's a great substitute for starchy grains like pasta and rice and is super quick and easy to cook. You can find quinoa in a variety of colors – the most popular are white, golden, red and black. To add extra flavor, cook it in vegetable broth and add some aromatic spices like smashed garlic, fresh rosemary, a pinch of sea salt, or fresh ground black pepper.

We recommend that you cook plain quinoa once in a while and store it in your fridge. You can add plain quinoa to ANY of the Operation Cleanse recipes during Vegan Detox and post cleanse or even add it to a soup for a "soupy rice" recipe!

Ingredients
1 cup dry quinoa
2 cups water or broth of choice

Directions
1.   Rinse the quinoa in a fine strainer under cold water for at least 2 minutes (this removes the bitter taste from quinoa's natural coating).

2.   Place quinoa in a saucepan with water. Bring to boil over medium heat.

3.   When boiling, reduce to low heat and cover until the water is absorbed (about 15 minutes). Do not stir the quinoa until liquid is fully absorbed.

4.   Once liquid is absorbed, remove lid and fluff the quinoa with a fork. You will see white rings forming when it's cooked. If you like it fluffier, add a few tablespoons of water and cook longer until water is absorbed.

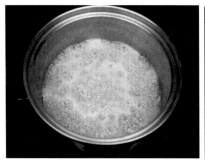 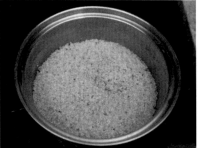 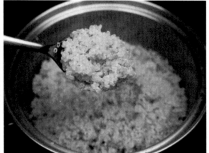

here's a *tip!*

If you need to cook more quinoa, follow the 2:1 liquid to quinoa ratio. Cooked quinoa can be kept in fridge for 2-3 days or frozen in cup portions.

Quinoa can easily replace any rice dish you love. Give "Rice & Peas" a try with quinoa as your rice!

take a look at what else you can do with quinoa ...

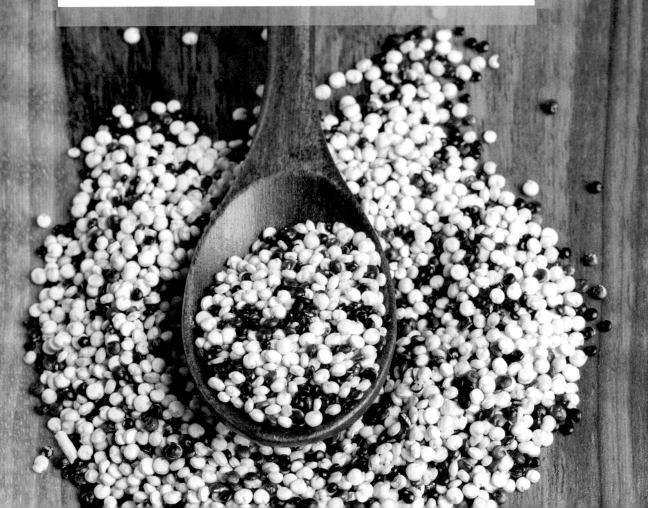

QUINOA SALAD WITH ROASTED RED PEPPERS, CUCUMBER, AND LEMON-HONEY DRESSING

Ingredients
2 red peppers, chopped
1 cup quinoa, cooked
1/4 teaspoon sea salt, or more to taste
1/2 ounce dill, stemmed and chopped
1 cucumber, seeded and diced

Dressing
3/4 cups lemon juice (2-3 lemons)
1 tablespoon mustard
2 tablespoons honey
1 ½ cups extra virgin olive oil
1 teaspoon sea salt

Directions
1.   Preheat oven to 375°F. Place peppers on sheet tray and roast until peppers begin to blacken and collapse, about 30-40 minutes. Transfer peppers to bowl, cover with dinner plate, and allow to steam 10-15 minutes. Skin and seed peppers and cut into medium dice. Set aside to cool.

2.   In medium bowl add cooked quinoa, peppers, dill, cucumber and toss to combine.

3.   In blender, combine dressing ingredients. Slowly drizzle in olive oil while machine is running until smooth emulsion is achieved. Toss salad with dressing to taste.

PINEAPPLE "FRIED" QUINOA

Ingredients

1 cup dry quinoa
1 cup low sodium vegetable
   broth
1 cup coconut milk
2 tablespoons olive oil
1 tablespoon grated ginger
1 stalk leeks, chopped
2 garlic cloves, chopped
1 cup peas, frozen
1 cup carrots, chopped
1 cup pineapple, chopped
2 tablespoons cilantro, chopped
3 tablespoons tamari sauce
1/2 lime

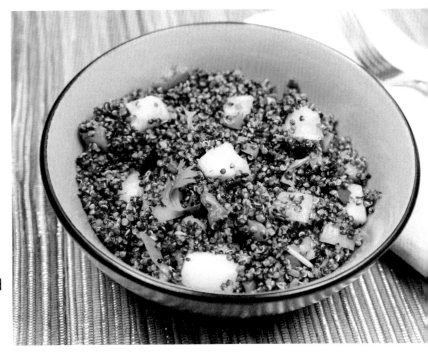

Directions

1.   Rinse quinoa and add to sauce pan with broth and coconut milk. Bring to a boil then cover with lid and lower the heat to medium-low until quinoa is tender and white rings form on the quinoa.

2.   Heat a separate skillet or large wok and add the olive oil, ginger, leeks, and garlic. Cook for 1 minute without letting garlic burn. Add peas, carrots, pineapple, cilantro and cook for additional 1-2 minutes until peas are tender.

3.   Combine quinoa with vegetables and pineapples. Add tamari sauce and lime.

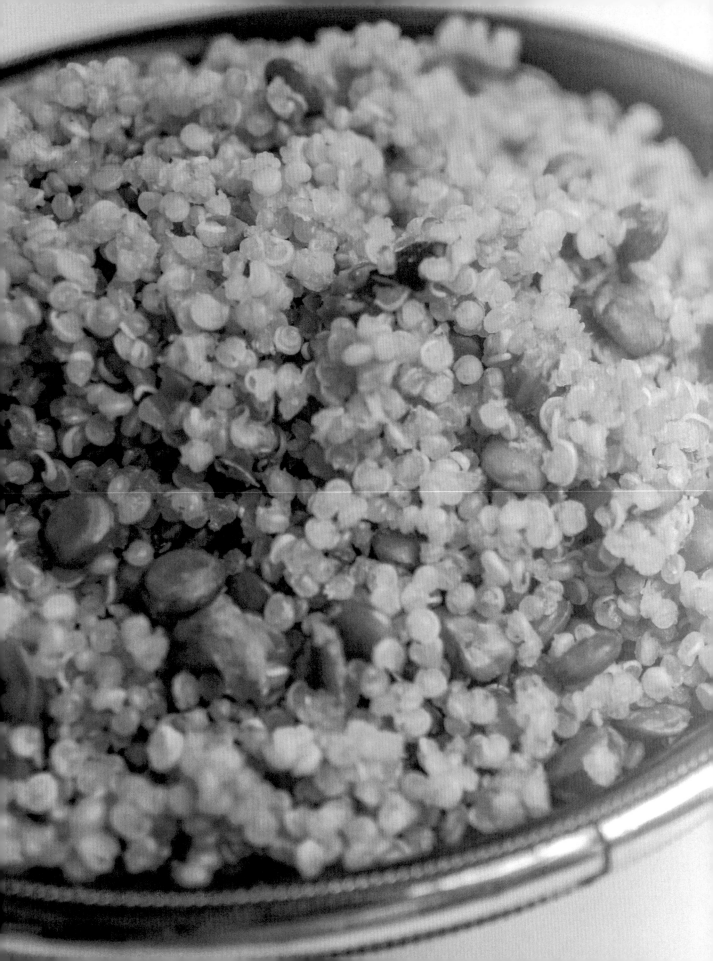

QUINOA AND LENTILS

Feel free to explore with this recipe. If you've made rice & peas in the past, you can make this!

Ingredients

1 cup dry lentils, rinsed
1 cup dry quinoa, rinsed
3 ½ cups water
1 teaspoon sea salt, or more to taste
3 tablespoons extra virgin olive oil
2 large onions (1 ½ pounds), sliced
8 garlic cloves, sliced
Fresh ground black pepper, to taste
2 lemons, cut into wedges for garnish

Directions

1.   In 2-quart pot, combine lentils, quinoa, water, and salt. Over high heat, bring lentils and quinoa to boil, reduce heat to low, cover, and simmer until all water is absorbed, approximately 30-40 minutes. Do not stir. Set lentils and quinoa aside with lid on to steam for another 10 minutes.

2.   While lentils and quinoa cook, heat oil in large sauté pan over medium heat. Add onions. Lower heat and cook onions until well caramelized, 20-25 minutes, stirring occasionally to prevent burning. Add garlic and cook for 2 more minutes.

3.   To serve, combine lentils, quinoa, and onion-garlic mixture. Season with salt and pepper. Garnish with lemon wedges.

4.   Serve with greens, or roasted veggies of choice. Great to top with the Cashew Yogurt recipe on page 92.

SIMPLE LENTIL SOUP

Ingredients
2 tablespoons extra virgin olive oil
1 large onion, diced
5 ½ cups of water
2 celery stalks, diced
1 large carrot, diced
3/4 teaspoon dried thyme
3/4 teaspoon dried basil
3/4 teaspoon dried oregano
3 cloves of garlic, minced
1 cup dry lentils
1 teaspoon sea salt
1/2 pound spinach, chopped

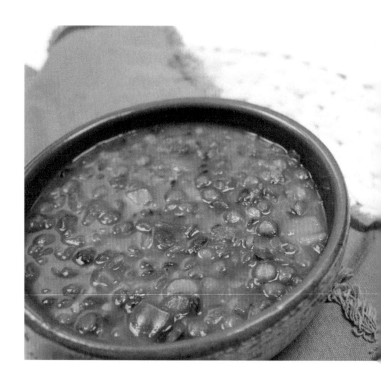

Directions
1.   Heat the oil in a medium size soup pot and sauté the onion until translucent. Add the celery and carrot and cook another 3-5 minutes.

2.   Add the thyme, basil, oregano, garlic, lentils and water.

3.   Bring to a boil, cover, and simmer until beans are creamy, about 30 minutes. Add more water if necessary, to desired consistency.

4.   Add salt to taste and spinach. Adjust seasoning if needed.

SWEET POTATO, KALE AND PUMPKIN SEED SALAD

Ingredients
1 sweet potato, cut into cubes
2 cups kale, chopped
1/4 cup pumpkin seed (can use any seed)
1 yellow pepper, chopped
1/2 onion, (optional)
5 tablespoons extra virgin olive oil
Sea saltand pepper, to taste

Directions
1.   Preheat oven to 350°F. Toss sweet potato and yellow pepper with 3 tablespoons of olive oil and salt and pepper to taste. Lay out on baking dish and roast until potato is tender.

2.   In bowl, mix kale and remaining olive oil. Massage generously. Add more olive oil if needed to soften the kale.

3.   Lightly sauté onion in 1 teaspoon of olive oil. Until fragrant.

4.   Mix potato, pepper and onions and transfer to bowl with kale.

5.   Top with nuts of choice.

Dressing
Top with balsamic vinegar or olive oil and vinegar.

BLACK BEAN AND SWEET POTATO SALAD

Ingredients
1 can low sodium black beans, rinsed, drained
1 sweet potato, cubed
1/2 tablespoon sea salt, or more to taste
1 tablespoon extra virgin olive oil

Optional Add Ons
Roasted cherry tomatoes
Roasted sweet potatoes
Sautéed onions
Sautéed zucchini
Toasted pumpkin seeds
Toasted almonds
Lemon zest and/or juice
Extra virgin olive oil
Chopped parsley or cilantro
Avocado

Directions
1. Preheat oven to 350°F.

2. Toss sweet potatoes in olive oil and salt to taste. Roast until tender.

3. Combine beans with roasted sweet potato.

4. Add the embellishments of your choice, adjusting quantities to get the flavor and balance you desire. If you like, garnish with chopped cilantro, arugula, and/or sliced avocado. Serve warm or at room temperature.

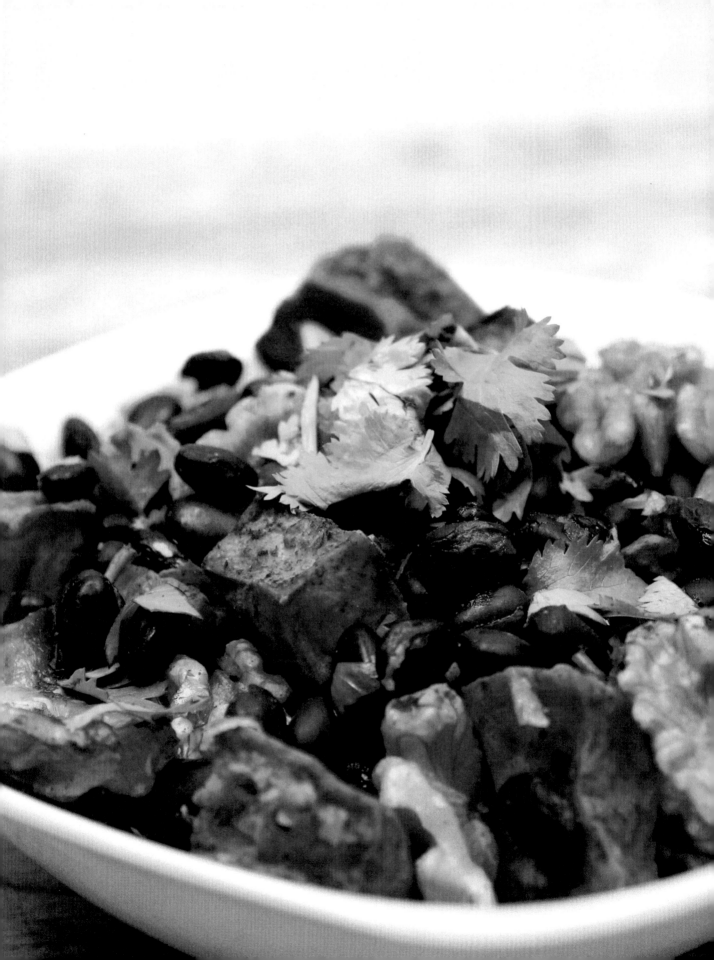

SPICY SWEET POTATO WRAPS WITH SIMPLE GUACAMOLE

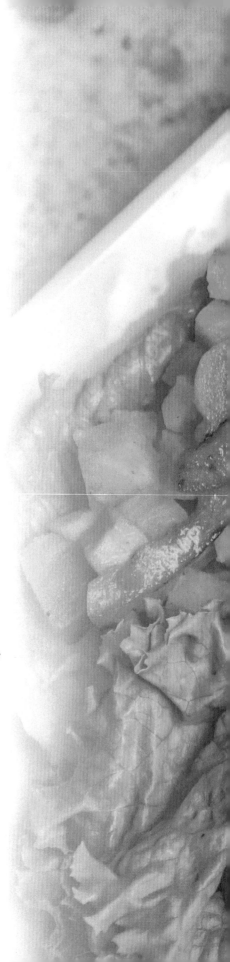

Ingredients

1 sweet potato, peeled and cubed
2 teaspoons extra virgin olive oil
1 tablespoon lime juice
1/4 teaspoon cumin
1/2 ripe avocado, pitted, peeled, cubed
1/2 cup tomatoes, chopped
1/4 cup onions, chopped
8 strips green peppers
Sea salt and pepper, to taste
Romaine lettuce (for wraps)

Directions

1.   Place cubed sweet potato in saucepan with olive oil, salt, pepper and just enough cold water to cover.

2.   Bring to simmer and cook until sweet potato is soft, about 10-15 minutes. Drain.

3.   Toss with lime juice and cumin. Set aside.

4.   Use fork to crush avocado. Squeeze additional lime juice over avocado. Add onions and tomatoes.

5.   Put wraps together. Top with guacamole and your choice of additional toppings.

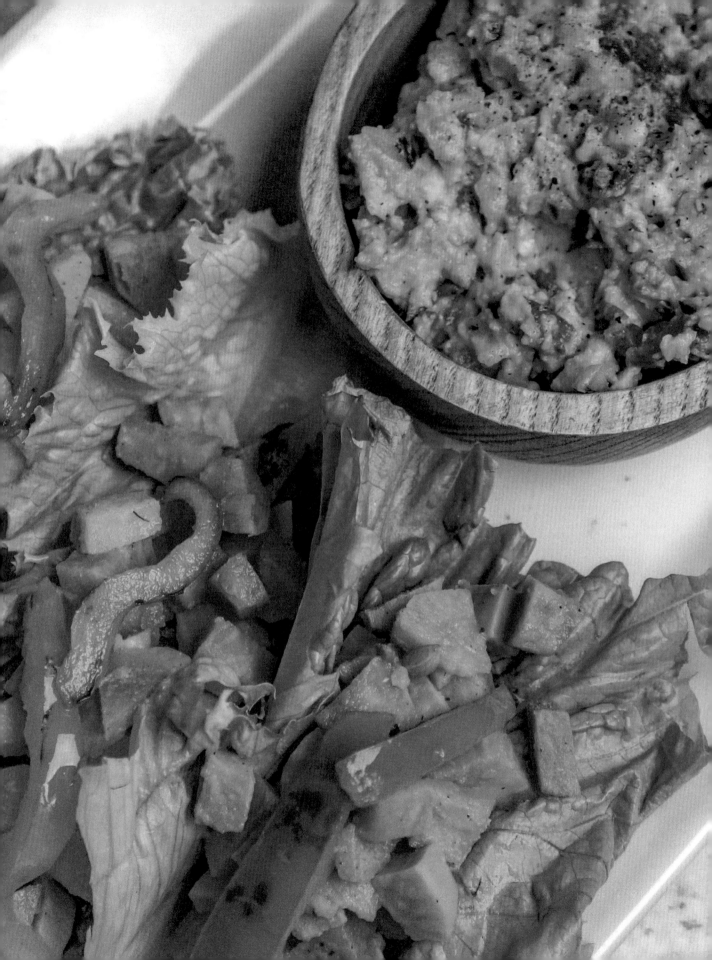

BEET MEDLEY WITH CASHEW YOGURT

Ingredients
3 medium beets, sliced into thin rounds
2 tablespoons extra virgin olive oil
1 teaspoon sea salt
1/2 teaspoon fresh ground black pepper

Cashew Yogurt
1/3 cup cashews, soaked 3 hours and drained
1/4 - 1/2 cup filtered water
1 tablespoon apple cider vinegar
1/2 teaspoon sea salt

Directions
1. Preheat oven to 350°F.

2. Toss beet rounds in olive oil, salt, and pepper and roast on a parchment-lined sheet tray for 20-25 minutes, or until tender.

3. Blend the cashews, water, vinegar and salt in a high speed blender until smooth, adding more water if necessary.

4. Serve over your choice of greens or quinoa and top with Cashew Yogurt.

Options
This also makes a great snack dish or you can serve with a side of additional veggies over your greens of choice to make it a heavier, more filling dish.

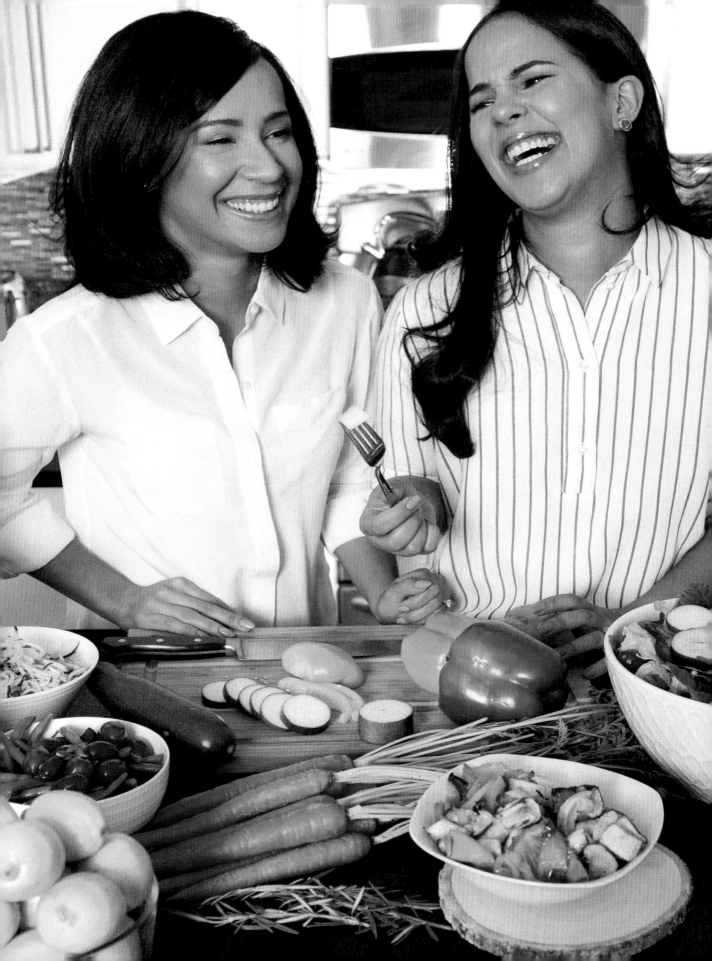

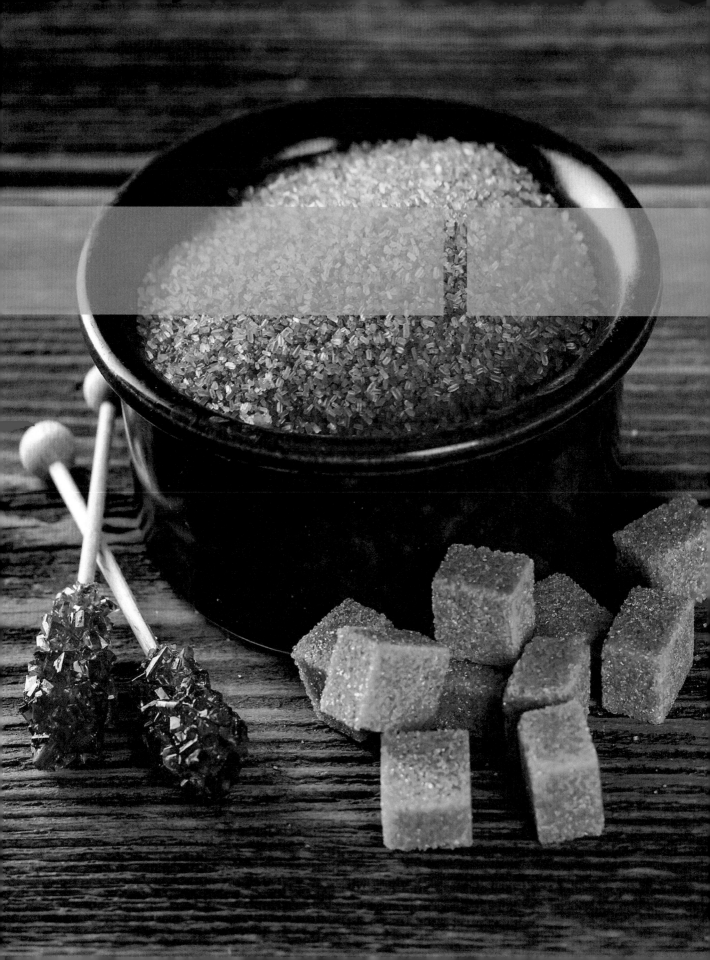

The Sugar Detox

LET'S KICK SUGAR TO THE CURB!

Are you ready to kick your sugar addiction? During Sugar Detox, get ready for a sweet treat - maybe not sweet, but definitely a treat! This week is all about eliminating sugar in every shape and form from your diet (no starch, no grains, no beans). Over the next 7 days, you are going to kick it up a notch with your greens and explore zoodle recipes. Once you choose your recipes, plan to add your choice of chicken, fish or turkey THREE TIMES during the week. Your serving size for animal protein is 4 ounces.

Want to kick it up a notch? Try going vegan during your Sugar Detox.

Note: The Sugar Detox recipes do not contain animal protein in order to give you the flexibility to add your choice to any of the recipes. Get creative with your spices and remember to shop organic as much as possible.

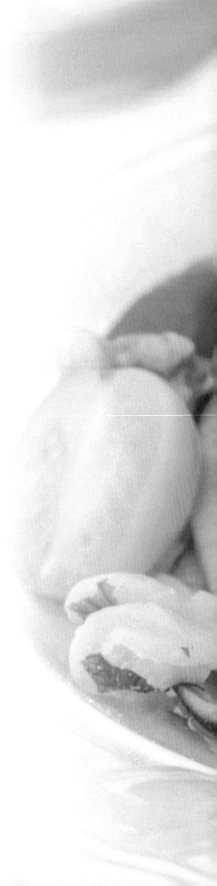

ZOODLE YOUR WAY TO WEIGHT LOSS

Serving Size
How ever much your heart desires!

We couldn't possibly skip adding the most amazing dish known to mankind ... zoodles (or zucchini cut into noodles using a spiralizer or a mandolin slicer).

This dish is great (and approved) during the entire cleanse. During Sugar Detox, add your favorite protein be it grilled chicken, grilled fish or even turkey meatballs. Skip the animal protein during the Vegan Detox and pack on all the veggies you want.

There really is no wrong way to make zoodles - as long as your sauce is homemade. Coming up is some *zoospiration*, let us see what you come up with using #OperationCleanse

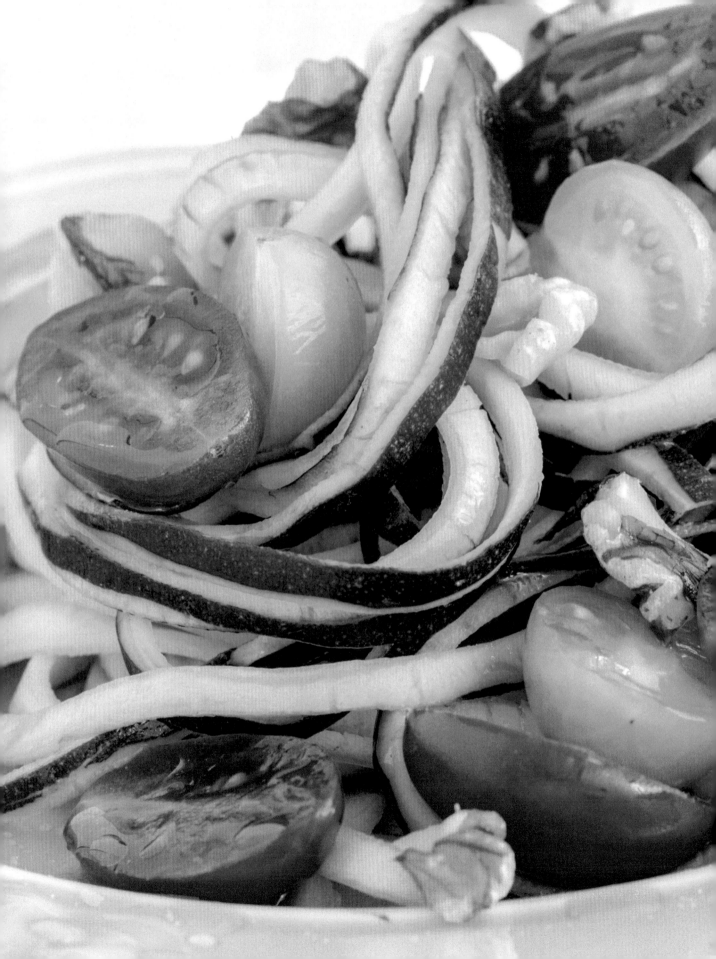

PEPPER ZOODLES

Ingredients
1 green pepper, diced
1 red pepper, diced
1 onion, chopped
2 garlic cloves, minced
Sea salt and pepper, to taste
1 zucchini, spiralized

Directions

1.   Sauté green and red peppers, onion, garlic, and salt and pepper, to taste.

2.   Add zoodles and sauté until combined evenly.

3.   Top with avocado.

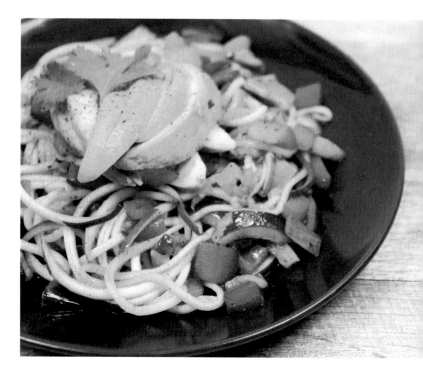

PESTO ZOODLES

Ingredients
1 zucchini, spiralized
Vegan Pesto, page 118
2 cups shitake mushroom
2 tablespoons extra virgin olive oil
Sea salt, to taste

Directions
1.   Preheat oven to 350°F.

2.   Toss mushrooms in olive oil. Salt to taste. Bake for 20 minutes until slightly crisp.

3.   Add 2 tablespoons of pesto to sauce pan and 1 tablespoon of olive oil. Stir lightly then add zoodles. Add more pesto to achieve desired thickness. Add mushrooms. Combine. Serve.

CHICKEN ZOODLE SOUP

Ingredients
2 tablespoons extra virgin olive oil
1 cup onions, diced
1 cup celery, diced
3 garlic cloves, minced
4 cans low sodium stock
1 cup carrots, sliced
3/4 pounds cooked chicken breast,
    cubed
1/2 teaspoon dried basil
1/2 teaspoon dried oregano
1 pinch dried thyme (optional)
Sea salt and black pepper, to taste
3 zucchini, spiralized

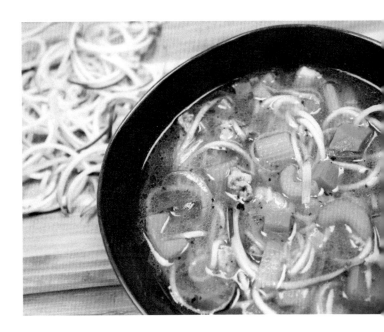

Directions
1.   Heat olive oil in a large pot over medium-high heat. Sauté onion, celery, and garlic until just tender. Approximately 5 minutes.

2.   Pour broth into the pot. Add carrots, chicken, basil, oregano, thyme, salt, and pepper. Bring the broth to a boil, reduce heat to medium-low and simmer mixture until the vegetables are tender. Approximately 20 minutes.

3.   Put desired zoodle amount into bowl and pour broth mixture over the zoodles.

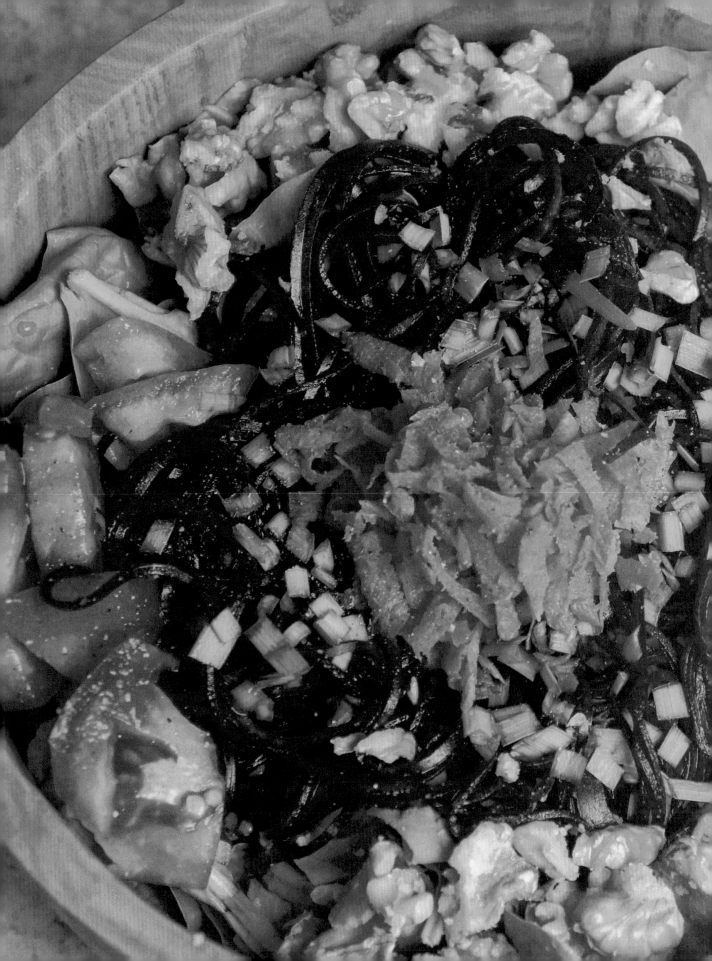

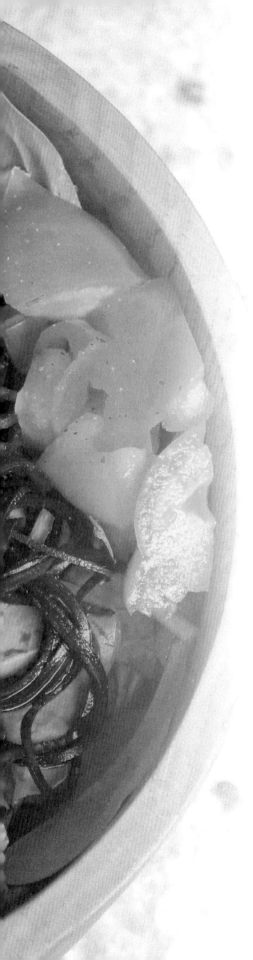

SPIRALIZED HERBED BEET SALAD

Ingredients
2 medium beets, peeled
1/3 cup freshly squeezed orange juice (about 2 oranges)
3 tablespoons balsamic vinegar
1 tablespoon tamari sauce
1/4 teaspoon sea salt, or more to taste
1/4 teaspoon black pepper, or more to taste
1 bunch chives, chopped
4 cups baby spinach, washed
Chopped walnuts (or any other nut)
1 tomato, chopped

Directions
1.   Cut beets into long strands by running them on a spiralizer. You can also grate on the large holes of a box grater.

2.   In a medium bowl, combine orange juice, balsamic vinegar, tamari, salt, and pepper and whisk to incorporate, and pour over beets then cover bowl and refrigerate for one hour.

3.   Before serving, toss with chives. Adjust salt and pepper to taste. Add tomatoes and nuts. Serve over a bed of spinach or any preferred leafy green.

SPICED CAULIFLOWER SALAD

Ingredients

1 large head cauliflower, chopped
1 tablespoon coconut oil
1 medium onion, finely chopped
2 green chilies, finely chopped (optional)
1-inch piece of fresh ginger, peeled and minced
1/2 teaspoon sea salt
1/2 teaspoon ground turmeric
1/4 cup water
1 handful cilantro leaves, finely chopped

Directions

1.   Place cauliflower in boiling water about 5 minutes.
Remove and drain.

2.   Sauté onion in coconut oil until onion turns
translucent.

3.   Add ginger and green chili and sauté for 2-3
minutes. Add cauliflower, turmeric, salt, and a little
water. Cover and cook on low heat until cauliflower is
warmed through.

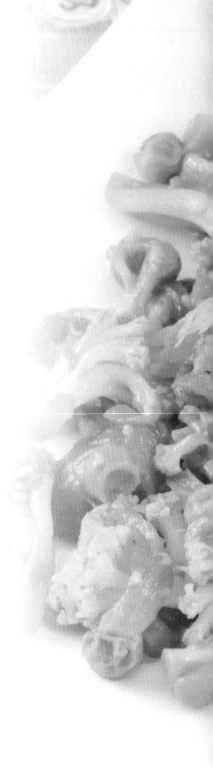

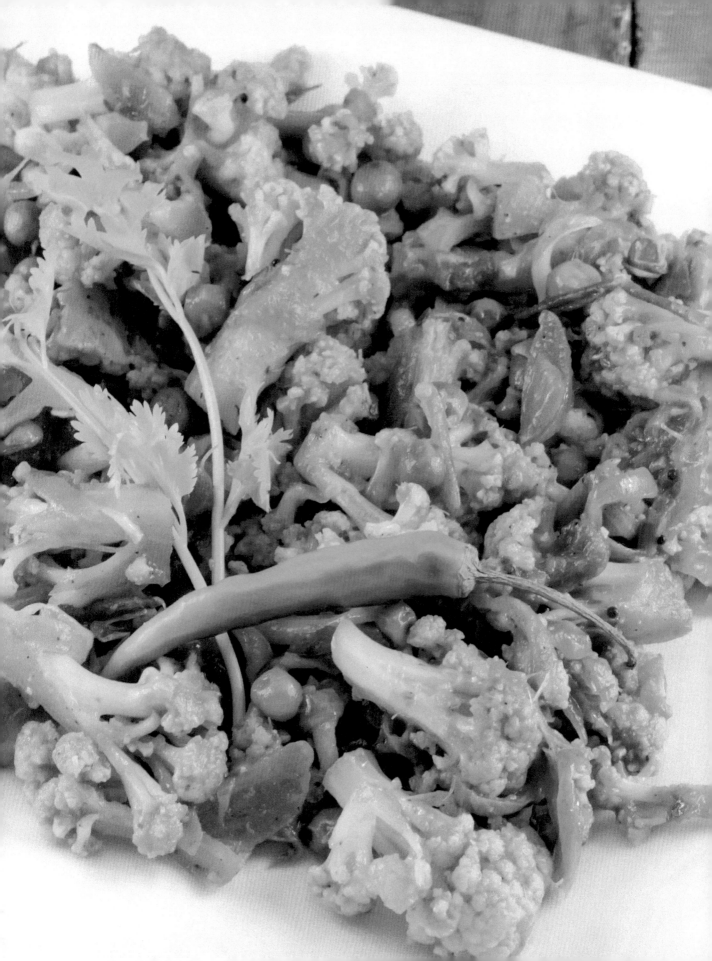

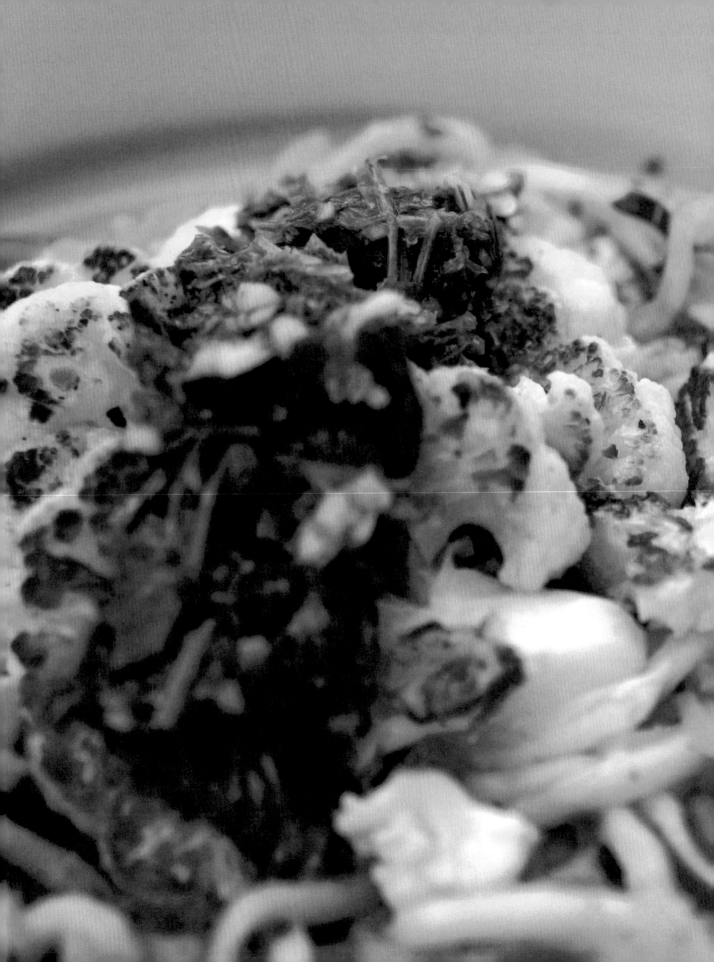

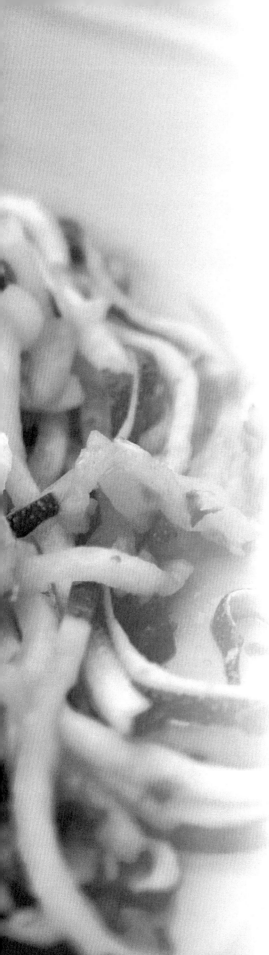

CAULIFLOWER "STEAK" WITH CHIMICHURRI

Ingredients
1 cauliflower head, cut crosswise 1/2 inch
1 tablespoon coconut oil

Chimichurri Sauce
1 tablespoon sea salt, or to taste
1 pinch of cilantro, about a nickel size
4 garlic cloves, minced
1 tablespoon apple cider vinegar
Red chili flakes, to taste (optional)
1/4 cup extra virgin olive oil

Directions
1.   Preheat a large deep sauté pan over medium heat. Add coconut oil and in batches sear the cauliflower pieces on each side (should take 2-3 minutes) season with salt to taste.

2.   Combine chopped cilantro, garlic, vinegar, 1 tablespoon of sea salt and red chili flakes in a food processor or blender and pulse until smooth. Slowly stream in the oil.

3.   To serve, drizzle chimichurri over the cauliflower. Pictured with garlic and tamari sautéed zoodles.

ZUCCHINI RAVIOLI

Ingredients

1 pound lean ground turkey
2 tablespoons tamari sauce
1 onion, chopped
2 garlic cloves, minced
Oregano and cumin, to taste
Extra virgin olive oil, to taste
Sea salt and pepper, to taste
2-3 zucchinis, depending on size

here's a *tip!*

Go vegan! Stuff with sautéed tofu or a mushroom and spinach sauté.

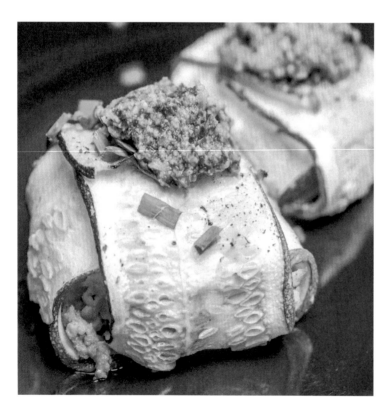

Directions

1. In saucepan, heat olive oil and add onion and garlic. Once simmering, add ground turkey. Add tamari, oregano and cumin to taste. Cook through.

2. Slice zucchini with peeler into strips. Lightly coat with olive oil and sprinkle salt and pepper.

3. Assemble ravioli using 2 strips and 2 tablespoons of turkey. Wrap and place face down on baking dish. Bake at 350°F for 20 minutes. Serve. Top with pesto on page 118.

SPICED TURKEY AVOCADO WRAP

Ingredients

2 tablespoons extra virgin olive oil
1 medium yellow onion, chopped
2 garlic cloves, minced
1-inch fresh ginger, chopped
2 large carrots, shredded
Cayenne and turmeric (optional)
Sea salt and pepper, to taste
1 pound lean ground turkey
1/2 cup low sodium broth
1/4 cup cilantro, chopped
1 ripe avocado
Romaine leaves for wrap
1/2 lemon

Directions

1. Sauté the onions, garlic, ginger in oil 3-4 minutes. Add carrots and turkey. Season with salt, pepper, cayenne, and turmeric to taste. Cook through.

2. Pour in the broth and stir until broth evaporates. Stir in the cilantro. Set aside.

3. Assemble the wraps together using the romaine leaves. Add avocado and lime to taste. This is a great dish to prepare ahead of time. Can use the ground turkey over a salad as well.

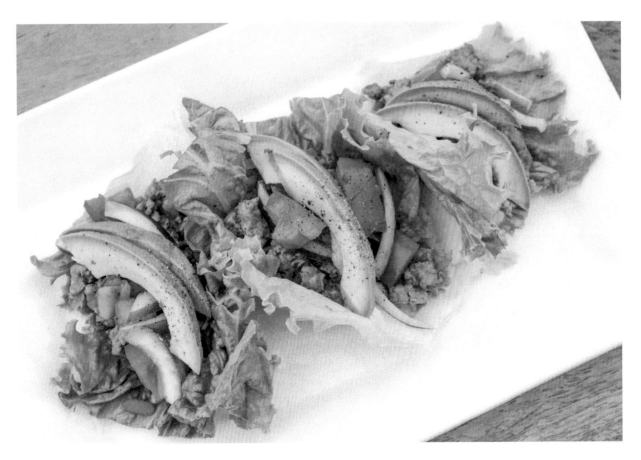

MUSHROOM PEPPER "STIRFRY"

Ingredients

1 box mushrooms (about 5 ounces), chopped
1 large green pepper, chopped in bite sized pieces
1 large onion, sliced
1 green chilli, slit
1 cup snap peas
3 garlic cloves, finely minced
1/2 inch ginger, finely minced
1 tablespoon lemon juice, to taste
3/4 tablespoons ground black peppercorns
2 tablespoons extra virgin olive oil
Salt, to taste
Tamari sauce, to taste

Directions

1.   Place mushrooms in salted boiling water for 2 minutes. Strain and pat dry with a clean towel and set aside.

2.   Add oil in a wok or heavy bottomed vessel. Once hot, add garlic and sauté for a few seconds. Add onions, ginger and chilli. Sauté. Add peppers and snap peas and sauté on medium-high for 4-5 minutes, tossing constantly.

3.   Add the mushrooms, place lid and cook on medium flame until soft and cooked. Stir once in a while. If there is any liquid, cook until the liquid is absorbed. Increase flame and toss. Add tamari to taste.

4.   Add ground black peppercorn and salt and mix. Turn off flame, add lemon juice and mix. Serve.

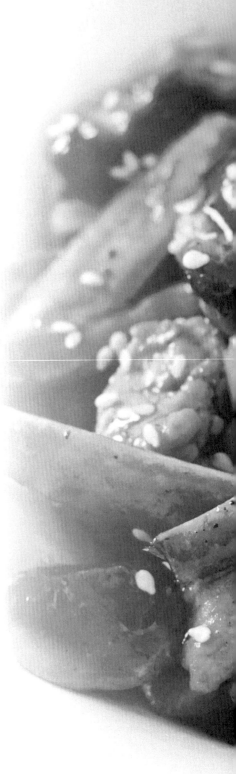

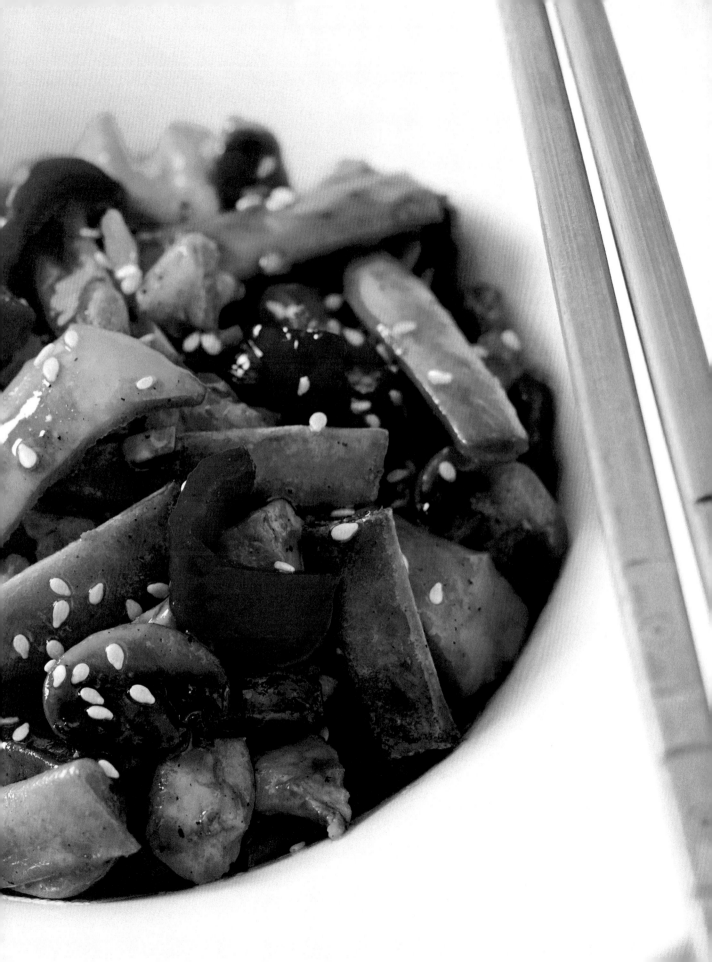

GRILLED ASPARAGUS WITH ROASTED ONIONS AND SHIITAKE MUSHROOMS

Ingredients
5 ounce bag pearl onions, root ends trimmed
1/4 pound shiitake mushrooms, stemmed and sliced
Extra virgin olive oil
1/4 teaspoon sea salt
1 bunch asparagus, trimmed, chopped to 1–2 inch pieces

Directions
1.   Preheat oven to 350°F. Combine onions, mushrooms, 3 tablespoons olive oil, and salt in a large bowl. Toss to combine.

2.   Transfer onions and mushrooms to parchment-lined sheet tray and roast until onions are caramelized and shiitakes begin to crisp, stirring occasionally. Approximately 30-40 minutes.

3.   While onions and mushrooms roast, preheat a grill (or pan). Toss asparagus with 2 tablespoons olive oil and 1/4 teaspoon salt, or more to taste. Cook asparagus until it takes grill form on all sides or about 5-7 minutes on a pan. You do not want to overcook. Keep the asparagus crunchy.

4.   When onions and mushrooms are ready, toss with asparagus and drizzle with Tahini sauce found in the Dips, Snacks and More section.

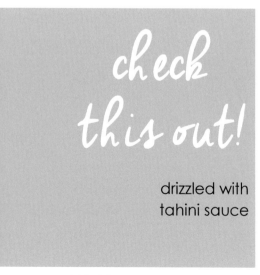

check this out!

drizzled with tahini sauce

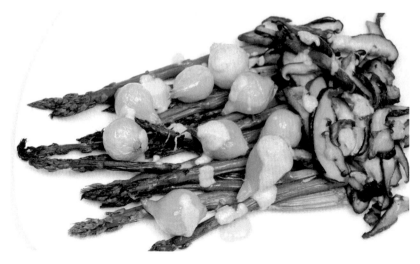

RAW CUCUMBER-AVOCADO SOUP WITH FRESH DILL

Ingredients

2 cucumbers, diced

2 avocados, pit removed and flesh scooped out

6 tablespoons lime juice

4 teaspoons garlic, minced

2 tablespoons extra virgin olive oil

1 ½ teaspoon apple cider vinegar

4 tablespoons coarsely chopped fresh dill

1 ½ cups vegetable stock

1/2 teaspoon sea salt

2 teaspoons red onion, minced

1 celery stalk, minced

8 sprigs of fresh dill for garnish

Directions

1.   Place 2 cups of the cucumbers, avocados, lime juice, garlic, vinegar, olive oil, dill, stock and salt into a blender. Blend until smooth.

2.   Pour mixture into a bowl. Add remaining 1 cup cucumber, red onion and celery. Stir well. Cover and refrigerate for 1 hour.

3.   Pour into serving bowls and garnish with a sprig of fresh dill.

CAULIFLOWER SOUP

Ingredients

1 tablespoon extra virgin olive oil
1 cup sweet onion, diced
1 cauliflower head, roughly chopped
2 cups low sodium vegetable stock
1 cup coconut milk
Sea salt, to taste

Directions

1.   Heat the oil in a saucepan and add the onion. Sauté until golden around the edges.

2.   Add the cauliflower and the broth to the pot. The broth should just cover the cauliflower.

3.   Simmer and cook until cauliflower is very tender, then transfer to a blender or using an immersion blender, blend until creamy. Add back to the original pot, and add coconut milk.

4.   Serve immediately with a drizzle of olive oil.

ZUCCHINI SLIDERS

Ingredients

1/2 pound ground turkey, chicken or beef
1 garlic clove, minced
1 tablepoon onion, diced
1/2 teaspoon sea salt, or more to taste
1/2 teaspoon ground pepper, or more to taste
1/4 teaspooon paprika, to taste
1 large zucchini
Extra virgin olive oil
Any other seasonings (optional)

Directions

1.   Slice the zucchini into quarter-inch thick circles. Drizzle oil over the zucchini and lightly pan fry. About two minutes.

2.   Combine the ground meat, garlic, onion, salt, pepper, paprika, and optional seasonings. Make small round patties same diameter as the zucchini slices. Pan fry the patties until cooked thoroughly.

3.   You can add additional toppings to your sliders, including tomatoes, avocado, mushrooms, onions, mustard, etc.

** For a Vegan Detox approved recipe, replace the turkey with chickpea meatballs.

ZUCCHINI AND TOMATO SALAD

Ingredients
1 zucchini, grilled and cut into half moon slices
1 tomato, chopped
1/2 cup onions, chopped
2 tablespoons balsamic vinegar
Sea salt and pepper, to taste

Directions
Mix all ingredients in large bowl. For variation, add vegetables from the approved veggies.

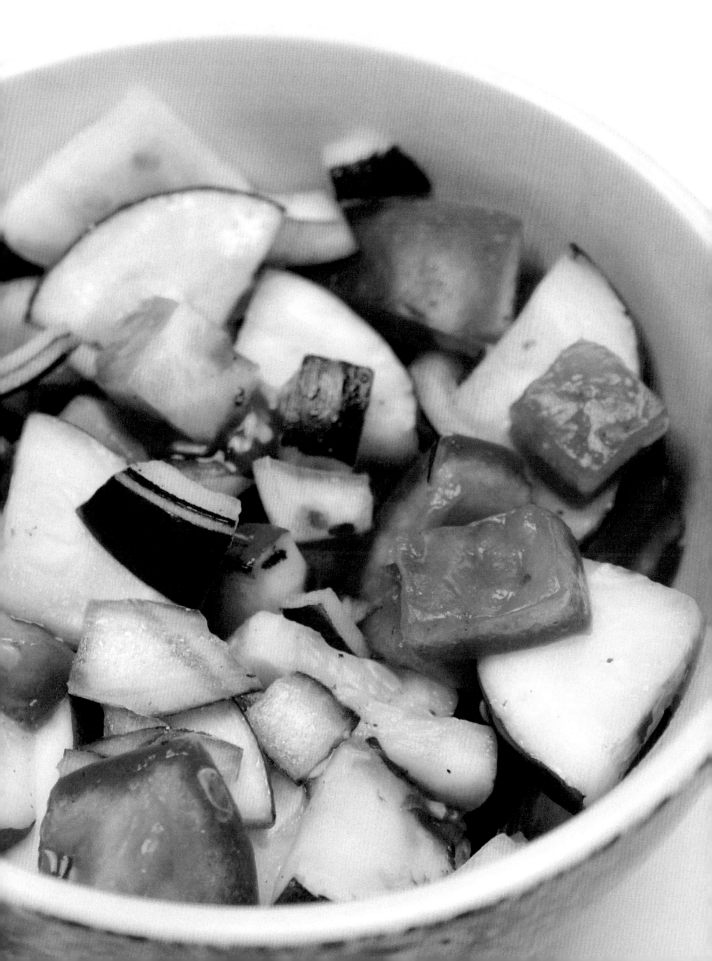

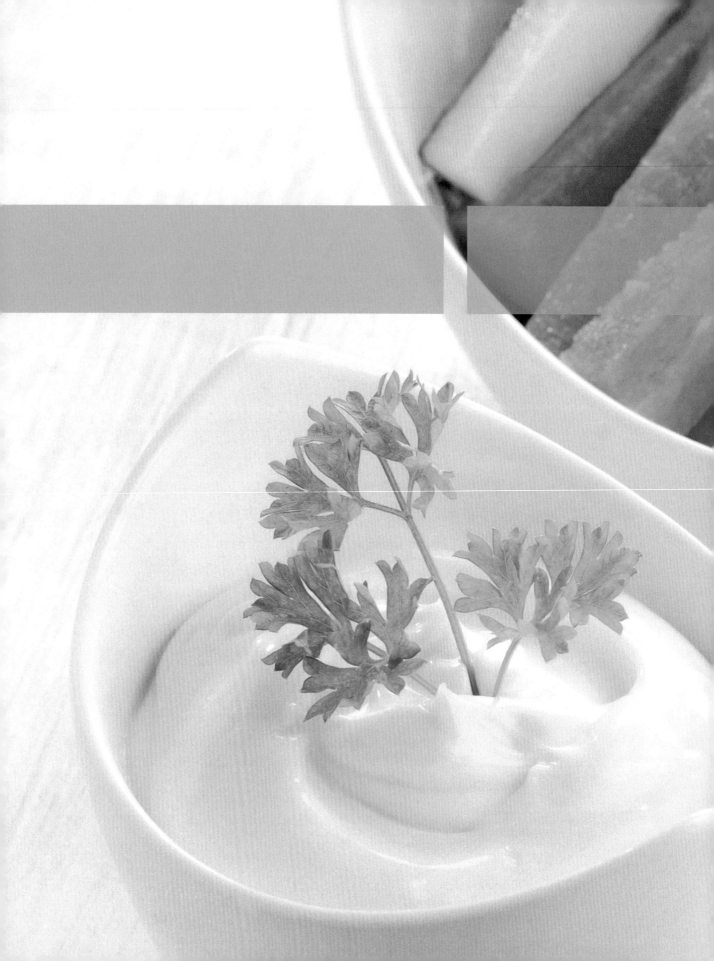

Dips, Snacks, & More

DRIZZLE IT OR DIP IT!

In this section you'll find delicious recipes for your morning and mid-afternoon snack as well as sauces for your vegetable sides or whatever your heart desires. If you're not following the sample menus we created, you must select 1-2 of the dip recipes for your mid-afternoon snack. If weight loss is part of your mission, the two daily snacks are an essential part of your regimen to help you achieve your goal – do not skip snack time!

TAHINI SAUCE

Ingredients
2 tablespoons tahini
2 tablespoons lemon juice (1 lemon)
2 tablespoons of water
1/2 teaspoon of sea salt, or more to taste

Directions
Whisk lemon juice and water into tahini. Add salt.

VEGAN PESTO

Ingredients
1 cup cashews
1/2 cup sunflower seeds
1/2 cup nutritional yeast
3 garlic gloves, chopped
1 teaspoon sea salt
1/2 cup water
2 tablespoons extra virgin olive oil
2 cups fresh basil

Directions
1.   Add all ingredients to blender adding the basil last.

2.   Blend all in a high speed blender or food processor. Add olive oil slowly as it processes.

3.   Store in an airtight container in the fridge and keep in mind that it will thicken as it sits.

Option: Remember, pesto serves as a dip and can be made with zoodles.

OLIVE TAPENADE DIP

Ingredients
2 cups pitted Kalamata olives
3 garlic cloves, minced
3/4 cups extra virgin olive oil
1/4 cup fresh parsley
1 teaspoon fresh thyme
1 teaspoon fresh rosemary
1/2 lemon, juiced
Fresh ground pepper, to taste

Directions
Place all ingredients in blender from lightest to heaviest. Blend until smooth.

CHERMOULA SAUCE

Ingredients
1 bunch carrot tops
1 bunch cilantro, stems included
1 bunch mint, de-stemmed
3 garlic cloves, minced
1/4 cup apple cider vinegar
Pinch of saffron
1 small jalapeno, minced (optional)
1-inch piece ginger, minced
1 teaspoon sea salt, or more to taste
1/4 teaspoon red chill flakes
1/3 cup olive oil

Directions
Place all ingredients in blender from lightest to heaviest. Blend until smooth.

Options
This sauce is great on ALL veggies, chicken, fish and yes, even tofu. Go ahead, get crazy and roast up your favorite veggies for a light snack.

SUN DRIED TOMATO DIP

Ingredients
1 medium to large tomato, cut into chunks
1 cup sun dried tomatoes
1 garlic clove, minced
1 tablespoon parsley, chopped
1/4 cup extra virgin olive oil
1 tablespoon nut of choice
Sea salt and pepper, to taste

Directions
Place all ingredients in blender from lightest to heaviest. Blend until smooth.

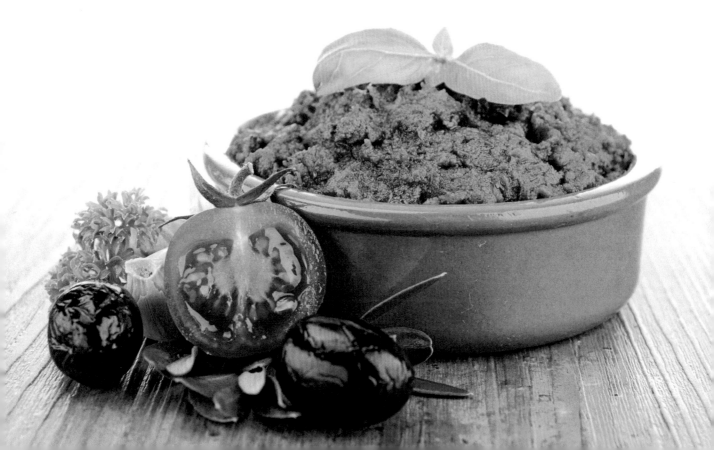

SPICY ROASTED TOMATO DIP

Ingredients

1/2 pound (about 2 handfuls) vine-ripe tomatoes, quartered
1 small onion, cut in eighths
2 garlic cloves, peeled
1/2 teaspoon chili flakes (optional)
1/4 tablespoon sea salt, or more to taste
3 tablespoons extra virgin olive oil
Fresh ground pepper, to taste

Directions

1.   Preheat oven to 350° F. Toss all ingredients in large bowl until evenly coated with olive oil.

2.   Transfer oven pan and roast sauce until all ingredients are well caramelized, approximately 30-40 minutes.

3.   Transfer to blender. Blend and puree until smooth.

4.   Add salt and pepper to taste.

AVOCADO CRUNCH

Ingredients

1 ripe avocado, diced
2 tablespoons sunflower seeds
1 tablespoon fresh lime juice
Sea salt and pepper, to taste

Directions

1.   Place all ingredients in a bowl and toss to combine.

2.   Season with salt and pepper to taste.

Options

Makes an excellent mid-afternoon snack.

CHIMICHURRI SAUCE

Ingredients
1 teaspoon sea salt, or more to taste
1 pinch of cilantro, about a nickel size
4 garlic cloves, minced
1 tablespoon apple cider vinegar
Red chili flakes to taste (optional)
1/4 cup extra virgin olive oil

Directions
1. Combine chopped cilantro, garlic, vinegar, salt and red chili flakes in a food processor or blender and pulse until smooth. Slowly stream in the oil.

recipe *ideas!*

Chimichurri sauce is a great addition for grilled veggies, grilled chicken, fish or even tofu if you want to go vegan.

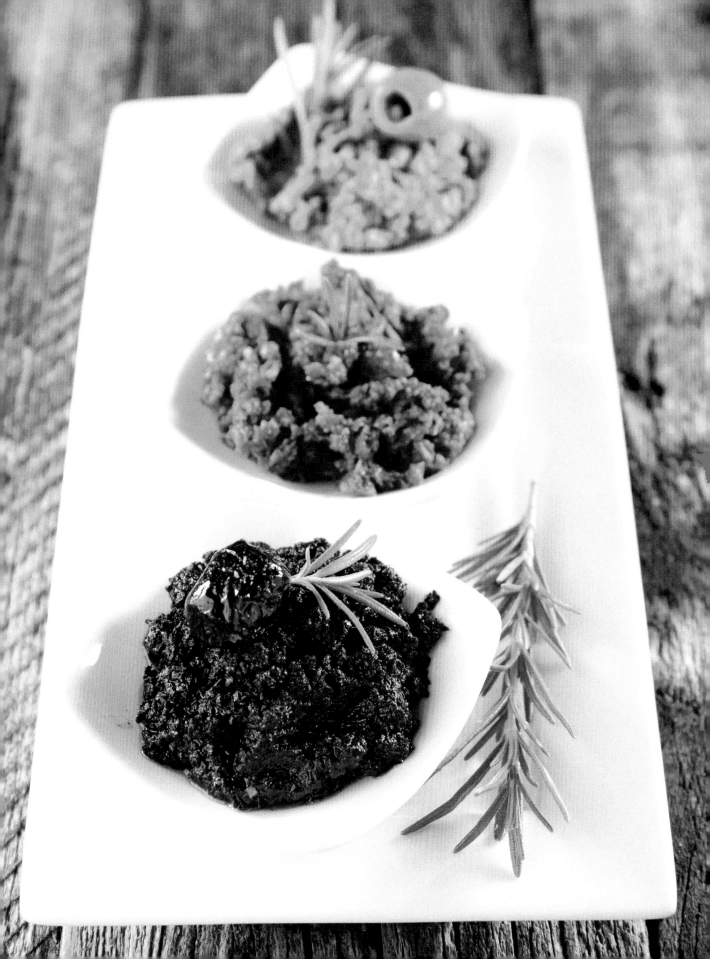

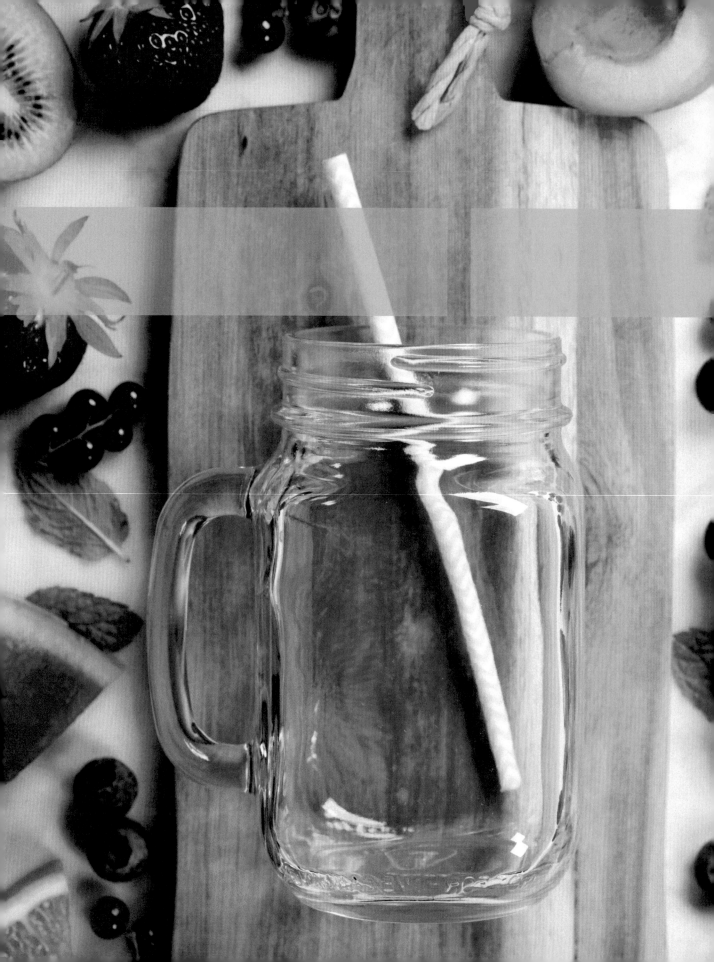

Smoothies

UNLESS OTHERWISE DIRECTED...

Simply wash and prep the ingredients as described, and then blend to perfection.

If you see coconut milk or almond milk, be sure to buy in a carton and not a can.

CANTALOUPE FLAXSEED SURPRISE

1 scoop vegan protein powder
1 ½ cup coconut milk
2 cups spinach
1/4 whole cantaloupe
2 tablespoons ground flax seeds

SWEET & SOUR

1 scoop vegan protein powder
2 cups kale
1 ¼ cups almond milk
1/4 cantaloupe
1 dime size of ginger
1 orange, peeled
2 tablespoons chia seeds

PEARY BERRY

1 scoop vegan protein powder
1 fresh pear, cut into chunks
3 strawberries
1 ¼ cup almond milk
1 small cucumber or 1/2 large one, chopped
2 tablespoons ground flax seed
quarter slice fresh ginger
a few shakes of cinnamon

APPLE RASPBERRY ORCHARD

1 scoop vegan protein powder
2 cups kale
1 cup almond milk
1 green apple
1/2 cup raspberries

BERRY PEACHY SURPRISE

1 scoop vegan protein powder
2 cups kale
1 ½ cup almond milk
1 cup strawberries
1 peach

PLUM FUN

1 scoop vegan protein powder
2 cups spinach
1 plum
1 peach
1 ¼ cup water
quarter slice, fresh ginger

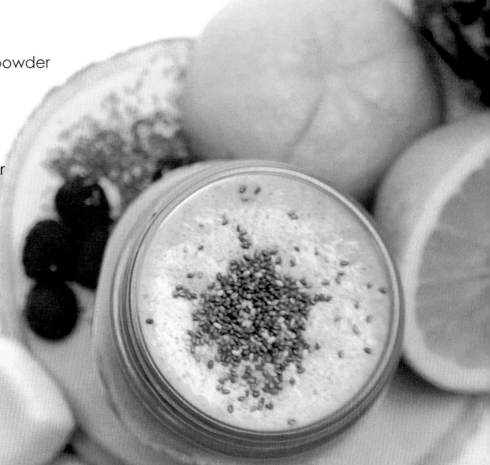

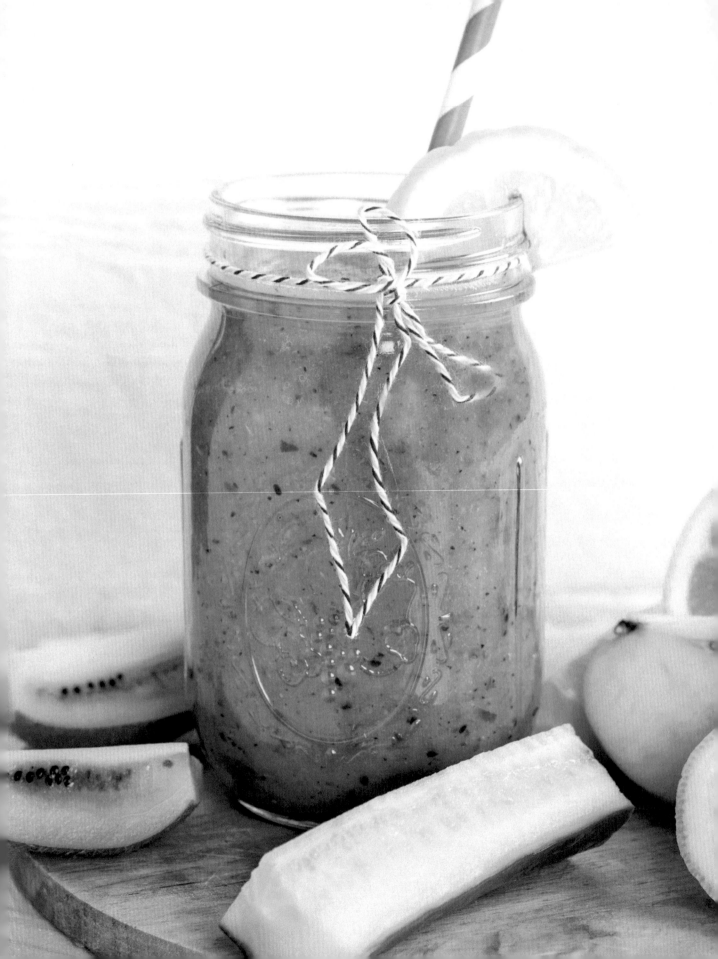

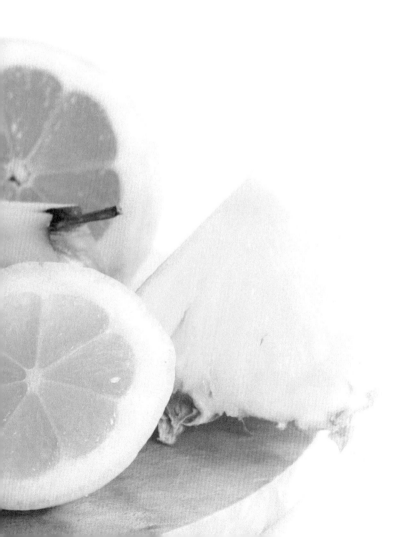

CITRUS SURPRISE

1 scoop vegan protein powder
2 cups kale
1 ¼ cup coconut water
1 cup strawberries
1 orange, peeled
2 tablespoons chia seeds

CITRUS DELIGHT

1 scoop vegan protein powder
2 cups spinach
1 ½ cup coconut water
1 orange, peeled
1/2 cup pineapple
2 tablespoons chia seeds

CUCUMBER SPICE

1 scoop vegan protein powder
2 handfuls of baby kale
1 ½ cup almond milk
1/2 cucumber, chopped
1/2 cup soaked raw almonds
fresh ginger, quarter slice
generous shakes of cinnamon
2 tablespoons of chia seeds

ALMOND RASPBERRY

1 scoop vegan protein powder
1 ¼ cup almond milk
2 cups spinach
1/2 cup raspberry
1/3 ripe avocado
fresh ginger, quarter slice
2 tablespoons ground flax seeds
1 tablespoon almond butter

BLACKBERRY-MELON DELIGHT

1 scoop vegan protein powder
1/2 cup blackberries
1/3 cup watermelon
2 handfuls of baby spinach
1 ½ cup almond milk
2 tablespoons chia seeds

SEXY CILANTRO

1 scoop vegan protein powder
1 cup almond milk
1 cup coconut water
1 cup papaya
1 cup cilantro
1 cup mango

here's a *tip!*

It's been shown that cilantro is incredibly detoxifying and can help pull metals from the body, so drink up, especially those of us who live in a city, have mercury fillings, or drink tap water!

VANILLA MILKSHAKE

1 scoop vegan protein powder
15 or so whole, raw cashews
1 tablespoon chia seeds
dash organic vanilla extract
dash cinnamon
1 ¼ coconut water
2 tablespoons ground flax seeds

APPLE PIE

1 scoop vegan protein powder
1 cup coconut milk
1 handful of spinach
1 small apple, cored and sliced
1 small slice of fresh ginger
1 teaspoon ground flax seed
generous shakes of cinnamon

PINEAPPLE CILANTRO DETOX

1 scoop vegan protein powder
2 cups spinach
1 ¼ cup almond milk
1/2 cup cilantro
1 cup pineapple
1/4 ripe avocado

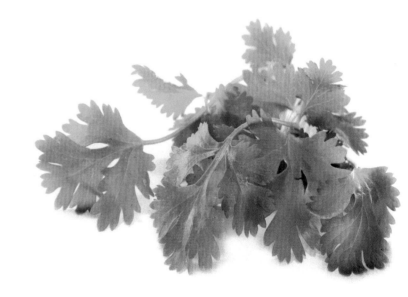

COCONUT DREAMS

1 scoop vegan protein powder
1 ¼ cup coconut milk
2 cups baby kale
1/2 cup mango
1/2 cup pineapple
2 tablespoons chia seeds

DETOXIFYING DANDELION GREENS

1 scoop vegan protein powder
3 cups dandelion greens
2 cups coconut water
1 cup mango
1 peach, chopped
2 tablespoons ground flaxseeds

on *dandelion*...

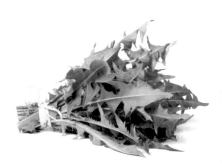

We know you mostly think of Dandelion as the pesky weed in your lawn. But Dandelion is a super herb that has great benefits on your digestive system because it is a pre-biotic (feeds the good bacteria). Dandelion acts as a mild laxative that promotes digestion and stimulates appetite. It can increase the release of stomach acid and bile to aid digestion, especially of fats. If you want to dilute its bitter taste, add a bit more fruit to your smoothie!

MANGO-BASIL HEAVEN

1 scoop vegan protein powder
1/2 mango
1/2 cup fresh basil leaves
1/4 juice of fresh lemon
1/2 cup spinach
1 ½ cup almond milk
cinnamon to taste

BASIL-LY DELICIOUS

1 scoop vegan protein powder
2 cups spinach
1/4 cup basil
1 cup coconut milk
1/2 cup pineapple
1 kiwi, peeled, chopped
2 tablespoons ground flax seeds

on *basil*...

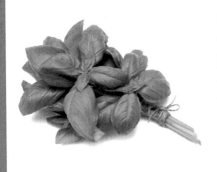

Basil is known as one of the worlds healthiest foods. Its benefits range from a super anti-inflammatory to immune-booster and cancer fighter! You can never get too much of it so, if your hand slips and you add more basil, it's ok! If you want to reduce the taste of it, just balance it with a bit of ginger.

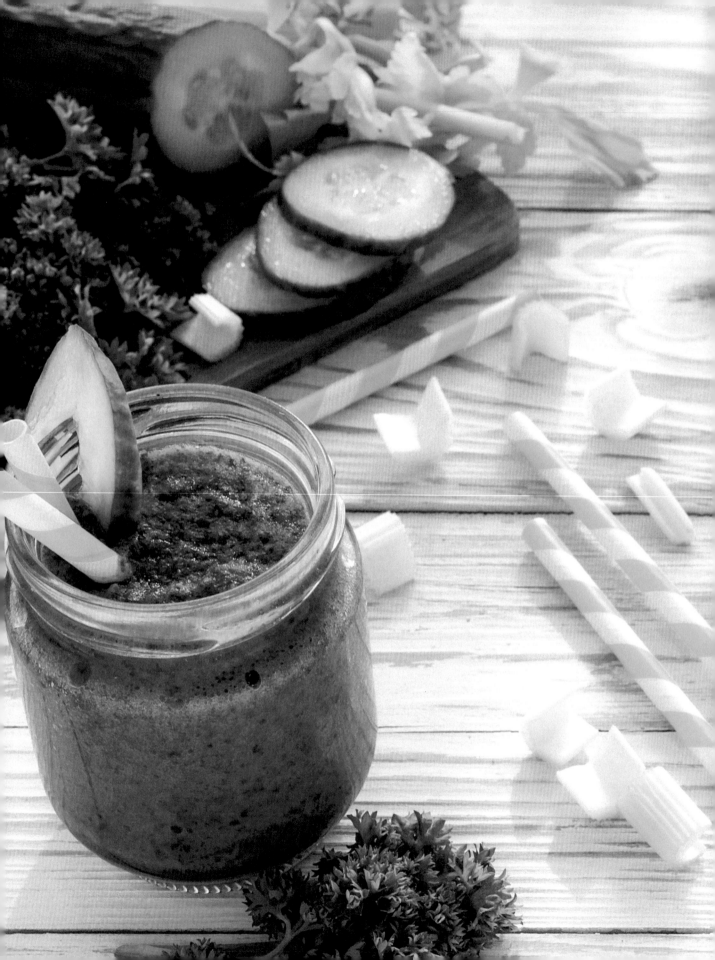

BEAT IT!

1 scoop vegan protein powder
2 cups kale
1 ½ cup coconut water
1/2 grapefruit, peeled
1 small raw beet, peeled and diced
(as small as possible for blending)
Juice of ½ lemon

SURPRISE GREEN

1 scoop vegan protein powder
1 cup spinach
1/2 cucumber
1 tablespoon lemon juice
1/4 avocado
1/4 teaspoon salt
1/2 teaspoon minced garlic
1 teaspoon olive oil
2 tablespoons parsley
water to desired consistency

ORANGE SORBET

1 scoop vegan protein powder
2 cups spinach
1 cup almond milk
1 cup papaya
1 orange, peeled
1 tablespoon chia seeds

PINEAPPLE CAKE

1 scoop vegan protein powder
2 cups spinach
1 cup almond milk, unsweetened
1 cup pineapple
5 strawberries
2 tablespoons ground flax seeds

BERRY FREEDOM

1 scoop vegan protein powder
2 cups kale
1 cup almond milk
1/2 cup strawberries
1/2 cup raspberries
2 tablespoons ground flax seeds

BERRY-PAPAYA BLEND

1 scoop vegan protein powder
2 cups spinach
1 ½ cup water
1 cup papaya
1 cup raspberries
2 tablespoons chia seeds

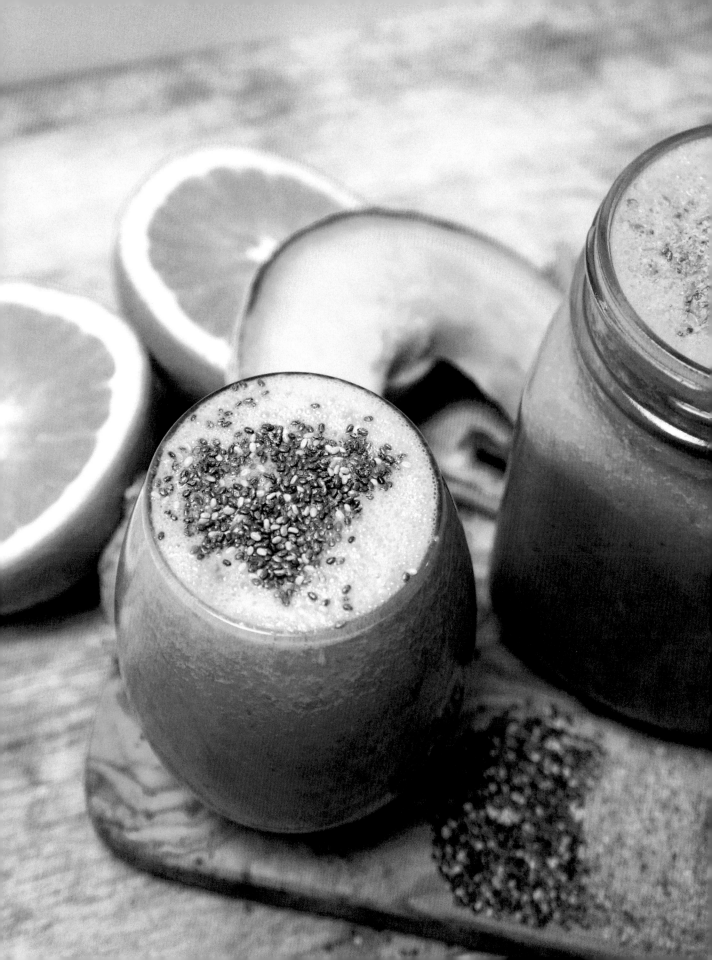

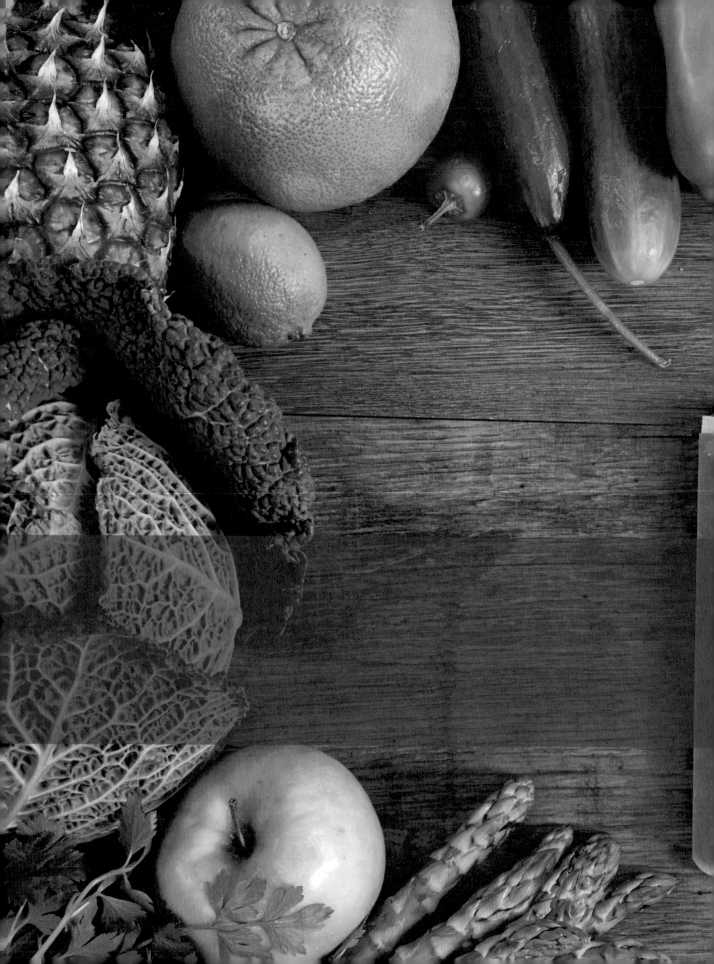

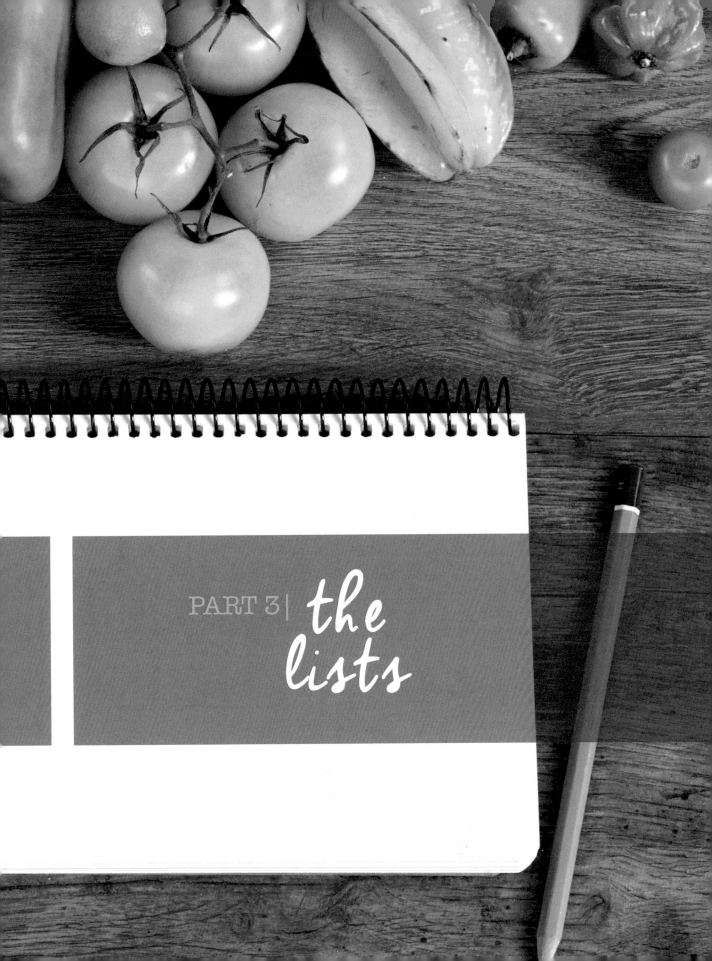

PART 3 | *the lists*

The Vegan Detox

7 DAY MEAL PLAN

	MONDAY	TUESDAY	WEDNESDAY	THURSDAY	FRIDAY	SATURDAY	SUNDAY
Breakfast Smoothie	Peary Berry Smoothie	Pineapple Cilantro Detox Smoothie	Peary Berry Smoothie	Pineapple Cilantro Detox Smoothie	Peary Berry Smoothie	Pineapple Cilantro Detox Smoothie	DIY* Smoothie
Mid Morning Snack	½ Cup Almonds	½ Cup Cashews	½ Cup Walnuts	½ Cup Almonds	½ Cup Cashews	½ Cup Walnuts	DIY* Nuts
Cleanse Lunch	Citrus Beet Salad + 5 Chickpea Balls	Sweet Potato Wrap + 2 Chickpea Balls	Pineapple Fried Quinoa	Citrus Beet Salad + 5 Chickpea Balls	Sweet Potato Wrap + 2 Chickpea Balls	Pineapple Fried Quinoa	DIY* Lunch
Afternoon Snack	Chimichurri Sauce + ½ Cup Carrots	Olive Tapenade + ½ Cup Carrots	Chimichurri Sauce + ½ Cup Carrots	Olive Tapenade + ½ Cup Carrots	Chimichurri Sauce + ½ Cup Carrots	Olive Tapenade + ½ Cup Carrots	DIY* Dip + Carrots
Dinner Smoothie*	Plum Fun Smoothie	Citrus Delight Smoothie	Plum Fun Smoothie	Citrus Delight Smoothie	Plum Fun Smoothie	Citrus Delight Smoothie	DIY* Smoothie

*If your goal is not weight loss, replace your dinner smoothie with any of the recipes from the Vegan Detox Recipes. DIY recipes are designed for you to use up whatever remains of your fruits, vegetables, lunch recipes, nuts and dips.

Vegan Detox Shopping List

PRODUCE

- [ ] Basil: 1 bunch
- [ ] Baby carrots: 2 pound bag
- [ ] Cilantro: 1 bunch
- [ ] Garlic: 13 cloves
- [ ] Green pepper: 2
- [ ] Leeks: 1 bunch
- [ ] Lemon: 5
- [ ] Lime: 1
- [ ] Onions: 2 (small)
- [ ] Orange: 2 (large)
- [ ] Parsley: 1 bunch
- [ ] Peas: 1 cup
- [ ] Pineapple: 1
- [ ] Red beets: 6
- [ ] Romaine: 1 bunch
- [ ] Sundried tomatoes: 1/3 cup
- [ ] Sweet onion: 1 small
- [ ] Sweet Potato: 3
- [ ] Tomato: 2 large

SEASONINGS

- [ ] Apple cider vinegar: 1 bottle
- [ ] Black pepper: 1 bottle
- [ ] Cumin: 1 bottle (powder)
- [ ] Nutritional yeast: 1 bottle
- [ ] Oregano: 1 bottle
- [ ] Red chili flakes: 1 bottle
- [ ] Rosemary: 1 tablespoon (fresh)
- [ ] Tamari sauce: 1 bottle
- [ ] Thyme: 1 tablespoon (fresh)

OTHER

- [ ] Almonds: 2 cups
- [ ] Cashews: 2 cups
- [ ] Chickpeas: 2 cups
- [ ] Coconut milk: 1 carton
- [ ] Egg: 1
- [ ] Extra virgin olive oil: 16 ounces
- [ ] Hemp seeds: 1 cup
- [ ] Kalamata (Black) Olives: 2 cups
- [ ] Low sodium broth: 1 carton
- [ ] Quinoa: 2 cups, dry
- [ ] Rolled oats: ¼ cup
- [ ] Walnuts: 1 cup

SMOOTHIE SHOPPING LIST

- [ ] Almond milk: 3 cartons
- [ ] Avocado: 1
- [ ] Cilantro: 1 bunch
- [ ] Cucumber: 3 (small)
- [ ] Coconut water: 1 carton
- [ ] Ginger: 1 small knob
- [ ] Kale: 2 large bags
- [ ] Oranges: 3 (large)
- [ ] Peach: 3
- [ ] Pear: 3
- [ ] Pineapple: 1
- [ ] Plum: 3
- [ ] Spinach: 2 large bags
- [ ] Strawberry: 2 large cartons
- [ ] Protein Powder

The Sugar Detox

7 DAY MEAL PLAN

	MONDAY	TUESDAY		THURSDAY	FRIDAY	SATURDAY	SUNDAY
Breakfast Smoothie	Very Berry Smoothie	Sweet and Sour Smoothie	Very Berry Smoothie	Sweet and Sour Smoothie	Very Berry Smoothie	Sweet and Sour Smoothie	DIY* Smoothie
Mid Morning Snack	¼ Cup Almonds ¼ Cup Cashews	½ Cup Pistachios	¼ Cup Almonds ¼ Cup Cashews	½ Cup Pistachios	¼ Cup Almonds ¼ Cup Cashews	½ Cup Pistachios	DIY* Nuts
Cleanse Lunch	Pepper Zoodles	Spiced Turkey Avocado Wrap	Pesto Zoddles + Ground Turkey	Pepper Zoodles	Spiced Turkey Avocado Wrap	Zucchini & Tomato Salad	DIY* Lunch
Afternoon Snack	Avocado Crunch	Sundried Tomato + Red Pepper	Avocado Crunch	Sundried Tomato + Red Pepper	Avocado Crunch	Sundried Tomato + Red Pepper	DIY* Dip + Carrots
Dinner Smoothie*	Orange Sorbet Smoothie	Pineapple Cake Smoothie	Orange Sorbet Smoothie	Pineapple Cake Smoothie	Orange Sorbet Smoothie	Pineapple Cake Smoothie	DIY* Smoothie

*If your goal is not weight loss, replace your dinner smoothie with any of the recipes from the Sugar Detox Recipes. DIY recipes are designed for you to use up whatever remains of your fruits, vegetables, lunch recipes, nuts and dips.

Sugar Detox Shopping List

PRODUCE

- [ ] Avocado: 3
- [ ] Basil: 1 bunch
- [ ] Carrots: 2 (large)
- [ ] Cilantro: 1 bunch
- [ ] Green pepper: 3
- [ ] Lemons: 5
- [ ] Onions: 4
- [ ] Parsley: 1 bunch
- [ ] Red pepper: 3
- [ ] Romaine: 1 head
- [ ] Sundried tomato: 1 cup
- [ ] Tomato: 4 (large)
- [ ] Zucchini: 6

SEASONINGS**

- [ ] Balsamic vinegar

OTHER

- [ ] Almonds: 1 cup
- [ ] Cashews: 2 cups
- [ ] Pistachios: 2 cups
- [ ] Coconut oil
- [ ] Ground turkey: 3 lbs
- [ ] Low-sodium broth: 1 carton
- [ ] Sunflower seeds: 1 cup

SMOOTHIE SHOPPING LIST

- [ ] Almond milk: 3 cartons
- [ ] Cantaloupe: 1
- [ ] Ginger: 1 small knob
- [ ] Kale: 1 box
- [ ] Orange: 3
- [ ] Papaya: 1
- [ ] Pineapple: 1
- [ ] Raspberry: 2 carton
- [ ] Spinach: 2 large bags
- [ ] Strawberries: 1 carton
- [ ] Protein Powder**

** You will have seasonings and protein powder left over from week 1.

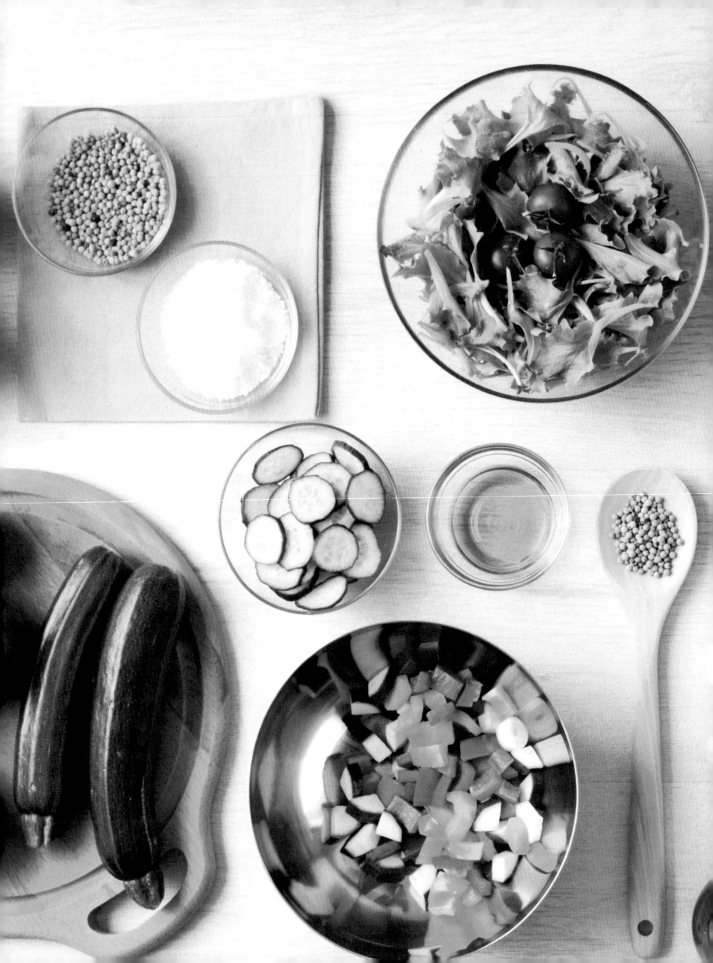

Getting Ready Checklist

START 4 - 5 DAYS PRIOR TO YOUR CLEANSE

1. Read ALL of Part 1 before you do anything else.
2. Purchase cleanse kit on OperationCleanse.com.
3. Start reducing coffee, processed food and sugar intake
4. Quit drinking alcohol TODAY!
5. Detox your kitchen! See "Getting Your Kitchen Ready"
6. Review the recipes and create your shopping list. Select 2-3 smoothies, 1-2 snacks, 2-3 lunch/dinner options and create your shopping list.
7. Take pictures and measurements! Record weight and measurement of arms, hips and thighs. Wearing a sports bra and stretchy gym shorts, take a picture from the front, side, and back. Remember to smile!
8. Clean your blender and set it on your counter.
9. Ensure you have sufficient food storage containers.
10. Review Kitchen Essentials List in Part 1 and purchase any items you don't already have.
11. Find a location to book a facial, massage, infrared sauna, or Colonic.
12. Find a certified colon hydrotherapists and book a colonic session. We highly recommend searching the referral database of International Association for Colon Hydrotherapy (i-act.org).

Food & Symptoms Diary

Many of us experience chronic headaches, migraines, bloating, gas and joint pains to name of few symptoms commonly triggered by food sensitivities. After completing the 14 days of Operation Cleanse, we encourage you to keep a detailed record of the foods you eat and symptoms they produce to help you recognize foods you are sensitive to.

Remember, there is a big difference between food allergies, food intolerance and food sensitivities. A food allergy is a dangerous, full blown allergic reaction in which your lips and throat swell up, to a point you cannot breathe. Usually you need a shot of epinephrine (Epi-Pen) to calm the immune system down. A food intolerance, like lactose intolerance is when our body lacks an enzyme to break down the lactose found in dairy. As a result, the bacteria in our gut tries to break the lactose down and produce symptoms from bloating and gas to diarrhea in some cases. A food sensitivity is neither an allergic reaction nor an intolerance. Certain foods or chemicals in foods cause our immune system to release chemicals that promote inflammation in our tissues and organs. Think of it this way, a very mild sensitivity that doesn't produce significant enough symptoms to cause concern multiplied by 365 days can produce the chronic symptoms that prevent us from feeling our best!

BASIC RULES FOR KEEPING A FOOD & SYMPTOMS DIARY

1. Write down everything you eat or drink, including all foods, beverages, supplements, vitamins, etc.
2. Be honest! You're only hurting yourself if you don't.
3. Write down the information as soon as you finish eating. It's more likely you will forget an item if you wait until later in the day or the next day.
4. Describe the type of food in as much detail as possible.
5. Describe how the food was prepared: raw, baked, boiled, steamed, etc. Also indicate if you followed any other special preparation or cooking techniques.
6. Use as much detail to describe your symptoms as possible. What was it? How severe? How long did it last?

DATE / TIME	SUPPLEMENTS	FOOD	SYMPTOM

Food Substitution Guide

As you review the recipes, you might find an ingredient you are allergic to, dislike, are tired of eating or simply can't find. Here is a handy list of substitutions you can use. Happy swapping!

INGREDIENT	SUBSTITUTION
ALMOND, FRESH	ANY OTHER NUT
ALMOND MILK	CASHEW MILK, RICE MILK
APPLE	ANY OTHER VARIETY OF APPLE, PEARS
APPLE CIDER VINEGAR, BRAGG'S	ORDER ONLINE
AVOCADO	ROASTED VEGGIES: EGGPLANT, MUSHROOM, SQUASH
BASIL	CILANTRO, PARSLEY
BLACK BEANS	ANY OTHER BEANS OR PEAS
BLACK-EYED PEAS	ANY OTHER BEANS OR PEAS
CANTALOUPE	HONEYDEW OR ANOTHER VARIETY OF MELON
CARROT	BEETS, SWEET POTATO, PUMPKIN
CAULIFLOWER	BROCCOLI, CABBAGE
CELERY	CUCUMBER, ZUCCHINI
CHIA SEEDS	FLAXSEEDS
CHICKPEA (GARBANZO BEAN)	GREAT NORTHERN BEANS, LIMA BEANS
CHIVES	SCALLIONS
CILANTRO	BASIL, PARSLEY
CUCUMBER	CELERY, ZUCCHINI
CUMIN, POWDER	CARAWAY SEEDS, CORIANDER POWDER
GREEN BEANS	PEAS
HEMP SEEDS	CHIA SEEDS, FLAXSEEDS, WALNUTS
KALE	ROMAINE, SPINACH, SWISS CHARD

INGREDIENT	SUBSTITUTION
LEEKS	CHIVES, ONION, SHALLOT
LIQUID AMINOS, BRAGG'S	ORDER ONLINE
NUTRITIONAL YEAST, BRAGG'S	ORDER ONLINE
OATS	BARLEY, BUCKWHEAT, MILLET
ONION	ANOTHER VARIETY OF ONION
ORANGE	CLEMENTINE, TANGERINE
PARSLEY	BASIL, CILANTRO
PEACH	APRICOT, NECTARINE, ORANGE
PEPPERS, FRESH	ANY VARIETY OF PEPPER
PINEAPPLE	ORANGE, MANGO
PUMPKIN SEEDS	ANY OTHER VARIETY OF SEEDS
QUINOA	ANY COLOR QUINOA
RADISH	RED CABBAGE, TOMATO
RASPBERRY	BLACKBERRY, BLUEBERRY, STRAWBERRY
RED LENTILS	ANY COLOR LENTIL OR BEANS
ROMAINE	SPINACH, SWISS CHARD
SHALLOTS	ANY VARIETY OF ONION
SHERRY VINEGAR	BALSAMIC VINEGAR, RED WINE VINEGAR AND RICE VINEGAR
SPINACH	ARUGULA, KALE, ROMAINE, SWISS CHARD
STRAWBERRY	BLACKBERRY, BLUEBERRY, RASPBERRY
SUN-DRIED TOMATOES	4-6 FRESH PLUM TOMATOES
SUNFLOWER SEED	ANY OTHER NUT OR SEED
SWEET POTATO	PUMPKIN, YAMS
TAMARI SAUCE	ORDER ON ONLINE
TOMATOES	ANY VARIETY OF TOMATO
WALNUTS	ANY OTHER NUT
ZUCCHINI	CUCUMBER, YELLOW SQUASH

Notes

Notes

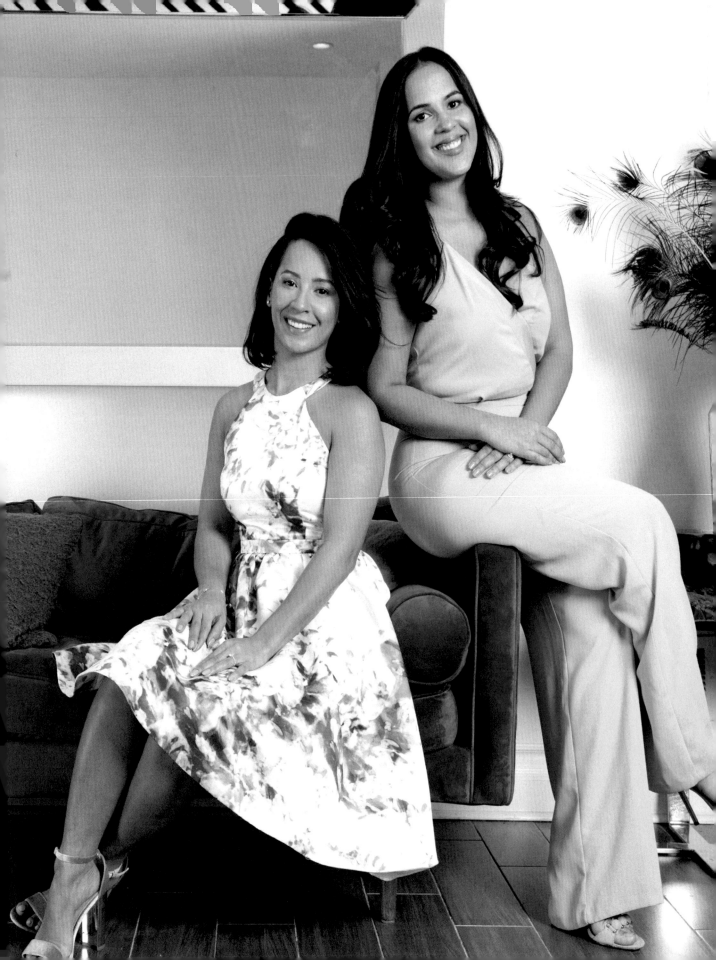

INDHIRA SANTANA

Indhira V. Santana is a leading bilingual nutrition & holistic health expert empowering women to find balance in their life and business without extremes. As a Latina and a thriving business owner, she teaches her clients to embrace the idea that you can be both fabulous and fulfilled in all areas of your life. She is best known for her practical approach to food, cleansing & healthy living and has built a successful holistic health spa franchise with her mother and sister in New York City called My Wellness Solutions.

In 2008 when she became a Certified Natural Health Professional (CNHP). Since then, she's coached hundreds to reach their health goals through customized wellness programs. In 2013, she graduated from the Institute for Integrative Nutrition (IIN), where she was trained in more than one hundred dietary theories and studied a variety of practical lifestyle coaching methods. Drawing on this knowledge, she helps clients create a completely personalized "roadmap to health" that suit their own unique bodies, lifestyles, preferences, and goals. She received her MBA from the Ross School of Business at the University of Michigan. In addition to public speaking she is a recurring guest on broadcast television.

VIOLET SANANA

Violet Santana, ND, CNHP is a Nutritionist who has helped many manage chronic illness including diabetes, PCOS, IBS, fibromyalgia, and infertility through her clinical nutrition approach and compassionate personality. She has dedicated her career to helping people achieve vibrant health through a combination of whole foods, herbs and evidence-based nutrition guidelines.

In her late 20's she became Certified by the International Association for Colon Hydrotherapy and has since administered thousands of colon hydrotherapy sessions where she taught her clients how to optimize their gut function. After completing her studies as a Certified Natural Health Professional (CNHP) and Doctor of Naturopathy (ND) at the Trinity School of Natural Health, she studied food and nutrition at a graduate level at the prestigious Columbia University. She is a frequent guest on broadcast television where she shares her expertise in digestive health.